Recent Advances in Imaging

(*Volume 1*)

Medical Imaging Technologies and Methods for Health Care

Authored by

Fuk-hay Tang

School of Dentistry and Health Science, Charles Sturt University, Bathurst, New South Wales, Australia

Recent Advances in Imaging

Volume # 1

Medical Imaging Technologies and Methods for Health Care

Author: Fuk-hay Tang

ISSN (Online): 2589-9414

ISSN (Print): 2589-9406

ISBN (Online): 978-1-68108-717-7

ISBN (Print): 978-1-68108-718-4

Published by Bentham Science Publishers – Sharjah, UAE. All Rights Reserved.

General:

1. Any dispute or claim arising out of or in connection with this License Agreement or the Work (including non-contractual disputes or claims) will be governed by and construed in accordance with the laws of the U.A.E. as applied in the Emirate of Dubai. Each party agrees that the courts of the Emirate of Dubai shall have exclusive jurisdiction to settle any dispute or claim arising out of or in connection with this License Agreement or the Work (including non-contractual disputes or claims).

2. Your rights under this License Agreement will automatically terminate without notice and without the need for a court order if at any point you breach any terms of this License Agreement. In no event will any delay or failure by Bentham Science Publishers in enforcing your compliance with this License Agreement constitute a waiver of any of its rights.

3. You acknowledge that you have read this License Agreement, and agree to be bound by its terms and conditions. To the extent that any other terms and conditions presented on any website of Bentham Science Publishers conflict with, or are inconsistent with, the terms and conditions set out in this License Agreement, you acknowledge that the terms and conditions set out in this License Agreement shall prevail.

Bentham Science Publishers Ltd.
Executive Suite Y - 2
PO Box 7917, Saif Zone
Sharjah, U.A.E.
Email: subscriptions@benthamscience.org

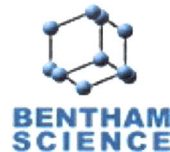

CONTENTS

PREFACE

The fast-moving advancement in medical imaging technology has revolutionized health care science. When information technology integrates with imaging technology, it is taking health care to new horizons. On the other hand, there is an increase in the number of health care workers to meet the need of growing population and requirement of quality health services. This accelerates the demand for applied and basic research on top of professional practices.

The potential and promising ideas in imaging technology are knowledge discovery and data mining in large image database, use of smart mobile devices in facilitating handy health care services, applications of biomechanical engineering methods and analytic methods for medical imaging. These thoughts are realized in the content of this book where it is divided into two parts. Part I deals with image management and knowledge discovery. It starts with an overview of recent advancement in Picture Archiving and Communication Systems. Then, the emerging mobile and cloud technology are discussed in Chapter 2. In Chapter 3, the applications of data mining and big data are explored.

In Part II, the medical imaging methods are extended for better health and disease detection. In Chapter 4, it high-lights the computer-aided method, while the recent study on the finite element analysis for breast image registration is elaborated in Chapter 5. Chapter 6 is a comprehensive risk analysis of Alzheimer diseases using image analysis while Chapter 7 examines bone mineral density evaluation methods by imaging. Lastly, Chapter 8 introduces how artificial neural networks work on skin lesions detection.

To meet the striking needs of this emerging discipline of health care science, the intended readers of this book are graduate students or researchers who are interested in research topics related to imaging technology. Also, this book will be of interest to health care community. It provides information for health care science and inspires new ideas for research.

ACKNOWLEDGEMENTS

I am greatly indebted to the co-authors who contributed to the chapters of this book:

Mr Edward Wong (Faculty Director - Medical Imaging Informatics, Hong Kong College of Radiographers and Radiation Therapists) helped me about the architecture and applications of the data mining program in Chapter 3.

Dr Janice Xue, my former PhD student and current research associate at the Chinese University of Hong Kong, wrote a detailed principle and application of biomechanical engineering method for breast imaging in Chapter 5.

Dr Christopher Lai of the Hong Kong Polytechnic University appraised the advanced imaging analytic tools for risk stratification of Alzheimer's disease in Chapter 6.

Dr Yau Ming (Patrick) Lai of the Hong Kong Polytechnic University and Professor Ling Qin of the Chinese University of Hong Kong reviewed the technique of bone mineral density detection using imaging and various methods in Chapter 7.

Last but not the least, Mr TT Wong, my former undergraduate student, and current practicing radiographer, carried out the experimental part of computer-aided detection for skin cancer detection and helped to prepare the manuscript in Chapter 8.

I thank all the above researchers by spending countless days and nights to the success completion of this book.

CONSENT FOR PUBLICATION

Not applicable.

CONFLICT OF INTEREST

The author declares no conflict of interest, financial or otherwise.

Professor Fuk Hay Tang
School of Dentistry and Health Science
Charles Sturt University, Bathurst
New South Wales
Australia
Email: ftang@csu.edu.au
Tel: +61 2 693 32980

Introduction to Recent Advancement in Picture Archiving and Communication System

Abstract: The recent developments of information technology have enhanced the Picture Archiving and Communication System. There are developments in mobile devices, cloud computing technology and intelligence method in the PACS. This chapter elaborates the advancement that has been made and explores their impacts.

Keywords: Advancement, Cloud Computing, Intelligent PACS, Thin Client, Picture Archiving and Communication System, PACS.

1. INTRODUCTION

With the advent of fast speed network and smart mobile devices, the speedy delivery of data and information has reshaped the healthcare services. Recent developments of Picture Archiving and Communication System (PACS) and cloud computing are renovating the practice of patient management. Undoubtedly the explosion of smart mobile devices applications (the 'apps') and Gigabit Ethernet and 4G wireless mobile telecommunication technology are the drivers for the advances.

2. WEB-BASED THIN CLIENT MODEL

The models of PACS architectures can be categorized into stand-alone model, client-server model, and web-based model.

For stand-alone model, the PACS workstations have large computing capability and are able to provide local storage (SCU storage service) and run image processing and 3D reconstruction locally without relying on network connection. The workstations usually required an UPS to sustain the stability of the system.

For thin client model, the clients reply on services provided by a centralized server through network connections. The clients usually have limited computing power and local storage. Most web-based computers or smartphones, handheld tablet PCs can access to the PACS to perform similar tasks as standalone PACS workstations. The thin clients usually do not need local installation of PACS application software to designated computers. There is no AE title or port number requirement for the PACS workstation. Instead, the software or PACS client program is accessible through the web. This offers a ready-on-line solution for user of PACS where the PACS can be accessible for registered users nearly anywhere in the institution.

3. USE OF MOBILE AND CLOUD TECHNOLOGY

"Cloud computing is a model for enabling ubiquitous, convenient, on-demand network access to a shared pool of configurable resource that can be rapidly provisioned and released with minimal effort or service provider interaction." (National Institute of Standards and Technology, [1]). It is comprised of 5 essential characteristics: on-demand self-service, broad network access, resource pooling, rapid elasticity and measured service.

The service model may include "Software as a service (SaaS), Platform as a service (PaaS) and Infrastructure as a Service (IaaS).

The deployment models are: private cloud, community cloud, public cloud and hybrid cloud.

Traditionally, IT supports are very important for PACS deployment. Maintenance of database and everyday QA for image transfer are daily work for PACS manager. With cloud computing, on-site IT infrastructure is minimal. Patient database becomes centralized and there is sharing of data across the hospitals and imaging centres. By using cloud technology, essentially there is no need to install the PACS client, or they just install the on-demand active x components.

4. INTELLIGENT PACS

As PACS has become an essential technology to manage digital images for the past 20 years, it offers a vast resource for knowledge discovery through image data that present in the digital images. On the other hand, computer-aided detection and diagnosis (CAD) exploits computing methods to extract quantitative information to enhance clinical management including diagnosis in a more efficient way. It must be clear that CAD is used as a tool to assist a doctor who takes the computer output as a second opinion. The final decision is still lying on the doctor who manages a patient.

Usually CAD is resided in a stand-alone workstation. In order to facilitate efficient detection of abnormality, the CAD server can be integrated with the PACS [2].

Undoubtedly, the integration of CAD in PACS workflow would streamline direct viewing of CAD outputs and utilizes the PACS database and enhances a more accurate and efficient diagnostic process. Huang [3] described three scenarios about the CAD-PACS integration using different editions of CAD-PACS toolkit. Also, the results of CAD were combined with the radiologist reports using DICOM structure report (SR) object.

A further extension of intelligent PACS is that the PACS –CAD can be deployed in the cloud environment. This enables a speedy and handy access to CAD service through the deployment of smart mobile devices. In the below section, we described the use of mobile devices (ipad, iphone, android smart phone and tablet) for PACS.

The following is a design of a cloud-based mobile intelligent system integrated with PACS. The whole computer-aided detection system is deployed in the internet (the "Cloud") and it provides computer-aided computation service and web services.

The cloud-based mobile intelligent system consists of three major components: 1. CAD component. 2. The Interface Service component, and 3. Web Service component. This is further discussed in Chapter 2.

The unique feature of PACS is that images are stored in DICOM (Digital Imaging and Communications in Medicine) format. A DICOM data file consists of image header, including imaging modality, patient details, space for report and reasons for the test; and the the image pixel data (Fig. **1**). Extraction of information in the DICOM header provides a resource for data mining. On the other hand, the deployment of PACS in a hospital provides a source of large volume of image data. This facilitate knowledge discoveries in PACS. The use of data mining in medical imaging will be discussed in the chapter that follows.

5. CONCLUSION AND REMARKS

The establishment of PACS has been revolutionized from high performance unix server with standalone workstation to web technology with thin clients and smart mobile devices. PACS is no longer confined to a single workplace but becomes available nearly everywhere. However, this raises the concern for security and patient privacy.

On the other hand, PACS is not just an image distribution management system but a means that can generate knowledge and facilitate clinical judgment.

```
                          Width: 256
                         Height: 256
                       BitDepth: 12
                      ColorType: 'grayscale'
                       studyDate: '20151223'
                     studyTime: '092001'
                     SeriesTime: '092844'
                AcquisitionTime: '092844'
                    ContentTime: '092846'
              AccessionNumber: "
                       Modality: 'MR'
                   Manufacturer: 'ESAOTE'
                InstitutionName: 'The Hong Kong Polytechnic
     University'
            ReferringPhysicianName: [1x1 struct]
                    StationName: 'E-Scan Opera'
                 SeriesDescription: 'Turbo 3D T1_1'
         InstitutionalDepartmentName: 'Dept. of Health Technology and
     Informatics'
                ManufacturerModel Name: 'E-scan'
                      PatientID: '2568.501499201'
              PatientBirthDate: '20150101'
                     PatientSex: 'F'
                    PatientSize: 0
              BodyPartExamined: 'WRIST'
              ScanningSequence: 'GR'
               Sequencevariant: 'NONE'
                    ScanOptions: 'PFP\PFF'
            MRAcquisitionType: '3D'
                   SequenceName: 'T3D T1'
                SiiceThickness: 1.1000
                 RepetitionTime: 40
                      EchoTime: 12
              NumberofAverages: 1
              ImagingFrequency: 7.6602
                  ImagedNucleus: '1H'
                     EchoNumber: 1
          MagneticFieldstrength: 0.1800
           SpacingBetweenSiices: 1.1000
                EchoTrainLength: 1
     InPlanePhaseEncodingDirection: 'ROW'
                      F11pAngle: 65
               PatientPosition: 'HFP'
                       StudyID: '501499200'
             FrameOfReferenceUID: '1.3.76.2.1.1.4.1.4.2568.501499369'
                    Laterality: 'L'
              ImagesInAcquisition: 52
         PositionReferenceIndicator: ' '
                  S11ceLocation: 22.5500
                SamplesPerPixel: 1
        PhotometricInterpretation: 'MONOCHROME2'
```

Fig. (1). DICOM header information.

CONFLICT OF INTEREST

The author(s) confirm that this chapter contents have no conflict of interest.

ACKNOWLEDGEMENTS

Declared none.

REFERENCES

[1]   Mell P, Grance T. The NIST Definition of Cloud Technology. The National Institute Standard of Standard and Technology 2011. Special Edition 800-145. p. 2.

[2]   Dubey RB, Hanmandlu M. Integration of CAD into PACS. *2nd International Conference on Power, Control and Embedded Systems (ICPCES)*.

[3]   Huang HK, PACS and Imaging Informatics: Basic Principles and Applications, 2nd Edition. John Wiley and Sons, 2010, pp. 807-859.

CHAPTER 2

Mobile and Cloud Technology Applications in Picture Archiving and Communication System

Abstract: In this chapter, a model of secured mobile system is described for image distribution in hospitals. In this system, it consists of mobile application server and mobile application client. The mobile application server communicates with hospital PACS and the client is embedded in the end-user's smart phone. The IMEI code of the mobile phone is sent by SMS to designated user to ensure security. The system can manage DICOM images with image processing capability with reasonable image quality. The mobile PACS demonstrates a model of using smart phone to improve the efficiency of health care services by speedy delivery of image information.

Keywords: Filmless, Health Care, Medical Images, Mobile Phone, PACS, Smart Phone.

1. INTRODUCTION

Digital technology has been widely used in medical field in the recent years with the advent of fast speed wireless networks and the deployment of cloud computing technology. The use of mobile phone for management of medical image distribution and the cloud computing environment in medical application with the integration to hospital Picture Archiving and Communication System (PACS) have been reported [1, 2]. On the other hand, cloud computing is a model for Internet-based computing which allows users to access service or applications from the Internet (the 'cloud') without the need to know or control the technology behind. The advantage of using cloud computing technology is that resources such as servers, software application, and data can be shared on demand [3].

In health care and medical areas, there are problems of resource allocation when implementing digital and filmless environment. In addition, maintenance of the computer system exerts another loading on health managers. It follows that cloud computing model offers a potential solution for health-care industry as it can alleviate the burden of resource-demanding computer facilities and infrastructure while it can keep health-care data updated. Applications of the Cloud computing concept can be found in health care and medical areas such as ultrasound [4],

Fuk-hay Tang

content retrieval [5] and genomics [6].

With the development of speedy wireless data network, mobile and cloud technologies offer promising solutions for efficient delivery of health care services. In the following discussion, we attempt to elaborate on two application models of mobile technology and cloud technology in medical imaging.

2. APPLICATION OF MOBILE TECHNOLOGY IN PACS

There were initiatives for handy access to medical images by personal digital assistant (PDA), window mobile or iPhone [7, 8] or iPad [9] or other mobile device [6]. In general, mobile devices should be used for image review instead of diagnosis. However, for imaging modalities such as Computed Tomography and Magnetic Resonance Imaging with lower image resolution, it was reported that the mobile handheld device could be used for diagnosis such as in coronary computed tomography with the high degree of accuracy [10 - 12].

In the Internet network, security and patient privacy are concerns for realizing mobile applications. In that case, a security enhanced-mobile phone system for the distribution of medical images is probably a solution for immediate access to CT or MRI images in medical DICOM format and ensures protection of patient data in public networks. The system needs to be applicable for any digital images that meet medical standard and interfaces with existing medical PACS in hospitals.

2.1. Design for Mobile PACS

One design of a mobile PACS is that it consists of client-free application server. The mobile web interface can run on iPad, iPhone, Android and Windows mobile device/tablet. The mobile web interface is written in C# using Microsoft Visual Studio 2008 and HTML5.

A user needs to be pre-registered in the mobile web server with his/her name with mobile phone number and International Mobile Equipment Identity (IMEI) code. When an image set needs to be received for the attention of a registered user, the images are sent from the imaging modality to the mobile application server where it will trigger a Short Message Service (SMS) message as a security token to the mobile phone of the user. The security token can allow the designated user to retrieve the relevant images. The images are needed to be "decoded" with the relevant patient ID and history. This information will be sent separately thorough another web service call.

On the mobile device side, the mobile application client is based on a web client that can run web browsers on different platforms, *e.g* . Internet Explorer (IE) on

Windows, Browser on Android, and Safari on iPad. Hence, no pre-installed client on the mobile device (smart phone or tablet) is required. There are several advantages for this design:

1. One program run on multiple browsers/platforms
2. No pre-installation is needed
3. The system can be modified on the developer platform rather on the client side
4. Deliver to the server once and will update all the client devices (thin-client)
5. Easy to manage and maintenance

The web-based client is capable of (1) handling communication with the mobile application server as well as handling for the secure communication protocol, (2) handling data encryption and decryption, (3) displaying images for the end-user to view the image, and (4) handling image processing job for the images being displayed.

2.1.1. The Mobile Application Server

The mobile application server is the core part of the whole system. It centrally processes those images imported, and provides various services to the mobile application clients. The mobile application server is composed of two sub-programs. They are the mobile application server core program and mobile application workstation program.

2.1.1.1. The Application Core Program

The mobile application server core program is composed of the image processor component, the file management component, the SMS service component and the web service component.

The image processor component is mainly for handling pre-processing for the images before sending the mobile application client. The file management component is for image data storage and retrieval. The SMS service component is mainly for sending SMS message, which includes record access security key or record token, to the target mobile client. The web service component is the counterpart of the web client component on the mobile application client, which is mainly for handling communication between the mobile application client as well as handling for the secure communication protocol.

2.1.1.2. The Mobile Application Workstation Program

The mobile application workstation program is composed of the image importer component, the image viewer component, and the file management component.

The image importer component is mainly for manual image import to the system by end-user in case of linkage between PACS server is down or the PACS server is out of control. The image viewer component is an image viewer for viewing or reviewing images imported. Lastly, the file management component is the component responsible for the file storage and the in-and-out tasks.

2.2. Special Security Consideration

Since the image transfer will involve real patient data, the following security considerations are used for this system:

- The mobile-PACS server and mobile PACS application will be deployed in a designated room/computer rack with password/key locked
- An external firewall to protect the server from attack from outside
- A firewall between the server and PACS to restrict the unauthorized access from the server.

Security of Server

- Firewall installed on server to block all ports except 8080
- Antivirus, anti-spyware software installed on the server
- Username/password to restrict user access to application server's O/S

Security of Mobile Phone

- Password-locked mobile phones
- Access the data with valid username/password plus captured IMEI codes of the phone and record access key sent in advance by SMS

Security of Data Access

- Using predefined user with valid username & password to access the web services provided by the application server
- Pre-registered mobile phone number to ensure dedicated SMS to be sent
- International Mobile Equipment Identity (IMEI) code to enhance user access in clinical application of this system
- Record access security token key (record token) sent through SMS to access record in the server
- The security token key will be removed after 48 hours, *i.e* . the security token key is only valid for 48 hours to further enhance the user access
- Cryptographic protocol (SSL) to encrypt data transferred to and from server in clinical application of this system

2.3. Image Quality of the Mobile Device/Tablet

The mobile device under test is an iPad which supports a resolution of 2048 x 1536 at 264 pixel per inch (ppi) and screen size of 9.7 in (24.6 cm) diagonal (LED-backlit multi-touch display with IPS technology). The chip of the mobile phone device is A7 chip with 64-bit architecture and M7 motion coprocessor (1.3–1.4 GHz ARMv8-A dual-core CPU). The mobile device is capable of displaying a typical single slice of CT image of resolution 512 x 512 pixels that have around 0.5 MB in size.

3. APPLICATION OF CLOUD TECHNOLOGY IN COMPUTER-AIDED DETECTION

The use of cloud computing can expand and extend computer-aided detection (CAD) system to the mobile technology as it allows a mobile device to perform computational demanding task of CAD by sharing the application in the cloud.

3.1. Design of a Cloud-Based Mobile Intelligent System

The cloud-based mobile intelligent system consists of three major components (Fig. **1**): 1. CAD component. It is a stand-alone component that can read DICOM CT images and output patent's likelihood of disease automatically. 2. The Interface Service component. This component communicates with CAD component. Its function includes queuing the requests, calling the CAD to perform its job, closing the CAD and getting the result. 3. Web Service component. It is for handling incoming requests from applications such as uploading DICOM image request and requests for stroke results.

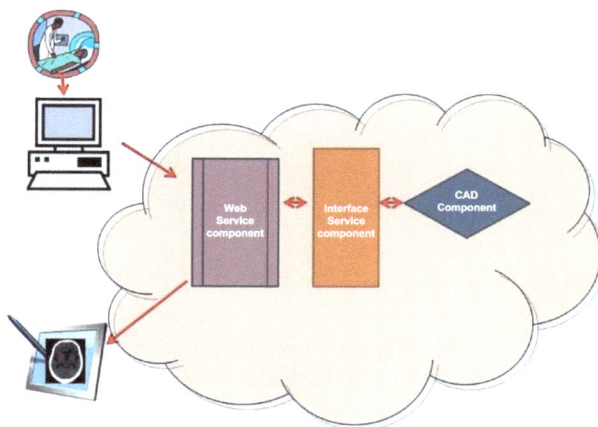

Fig. (1). Computer-aided mobile Cloud system.

The DICOM CT images will be retrieved directly from the PACS or from the user's DICOM workstation or mobile device and uploaded to the cloud-based mobile intelligent system, which returns the result of the estimated likelihood of diseases s to the mobile device. This will be handled by the client Web Service component and it can reside in different computer systems such as iPad, tablet PC, PC and mobile devices.

To improve the speed of image transfer, the LTE (**Long Term Evolution**) wireless communication is used to provide downlink peak rates of 300 Mbit/s, uplink peak rates of 75 Mbit/s.

3.2. Implementation Scheme

The programming language mainly used to develop the CAD Cloud system is C# and Microsoft Dot Net Framework 2. By using the C# language, we develop the web services. The web service is a set of web based functions which in turn will be used by any calling programs developed by other entities. The web services are running in the Microsoft Internet Information Service (IIS) which run on Windows Server 2003 or above.

For the application of computer intelligent system, we developed a computer-aided detection module based on our earlier works [13]. The CAD stroke module was developed by Matlab (version 2010, Mathworks, Massachusetts, U.S.A.) and was a standalone program.

4. DISCUSSION AND CONCLUSION

4.1. Security Consideration

Although mobile phone technology has become common in the medical arena, there are concerns about patient and data security. In our design, we proposed to use IMEI code registration method so that images would only send to the designated mobile phone and a one-off SMS activated security code ("the security token") for image retrieval. For the SMS token, it is only sent to the pre-registered users only. On the other hand, the IMEI code is sent to the server *via* HTTPS (*i.e* . SSL and thus it is encrypted). Also we can make use of remote data deletion services such as My Phone (http://myphone.microsoft.com) in case the mobile is lost.

4.2. Performance

As the design of the system adopts an open architecture, it is hence not solely dependent on a single type of network infrastructure. In principle, the mobile application client can use any kinds of network available on the mobile phone, such as 3G HSPA mobile-phone network, Wi-Fi (wireless network), second generation General Packet Radio Service (2G GPRS) mobile-phone network), and even Bluetooth network. It is expected that the 4G LTE advanced (Long Term Evolution Advanced) can reach the peak download speed of 1000Mbps and upload rate of 500Mbps [14] the outlook for application mobile and cloud technology in medical imaging is promising.

It is difficult to comment the overall performance of the mobile and cloud application as it depends on many determinant factors which may not be controlled by the end user, the developer and even the service provider.

The determinant factors of the overall performance of the mobile security system could be those listed, but not limited to, below:

The operating system and the system design of the mobile device

The CPU clock speed of the mobile device

The total and free memory available for the mobile

The bandwidth of the network

The actual traffics of the network in use

The number of routers/gateways involved in the whole system

The number of images transferred per case

The hardware and software configurations of the application server

The CAD cloud service does not need the users to control the technology infrastructure behind them. We proposed a private cloud implementation model but it can be extended further to public cloud.

CONFLICT OF INTEREST

The author(s) confirm that this chapter contents have no conflict of interest.

ACKNOWLEDGEMENTS

Declared none.

REFERENCES

[1]   Tang FH, Law MYY, Lee AC, Chan LW. A mobile phone integrated health care delivery system of medical images. J Digit Imaging 2004; 17(3): 217-25.
[http://dx.doi.org/10.1007/s10278-004-1015-5] [PMID: 15534754]

[2]   Law MYY, Tang FH. A scalable automatic bone age assessment system using the cloud computing technology for integration with PACS 19th Asian Australasian Conference of Radiological Technologists. Kaohsiung, Taiwan, China. 2011.26-27 March 2011;

[3]   Pallis G. Cloud Computing The New Frontier of Internet Computing. IEEE Internet Comput 2010; 70-3.
        [http://dx.doi.org/10.1109/MIC.2010.113]

[4]   Meir A, Rubinsky B. Distributed network, wireless and cloud computing enabled 3-D ultrasound; a new medical technology paradigm. PLoS One 2009; 4(11): e7974.
        [http://dx.doi.org/10.1371/journal.pone.0007974] [PMID: 19936236]

[5]   Town C, Harrison K. Large-scale grid computing for content-based image retrieval. Aslib Proc 2010; 438-46.
        [http://dx.doi.org/10.1108/00012531011074681]

[6]   Wall DP, Kudtarkar P, Fusaro VA, Pivovarov R, Patil P, Tonellato PJ. Cloud computing for comparative genomics. BMC Bioinformatics 2010; 11: 259.
        [http://dx.doi.org/10.1186/1471-2105-11-259] [PMID: 20482786]

[7]   Zeng H, Wu S, *et al.* An iPhone-based tele-health system for hypertension management. Int J Cardiol 2009; S128-8.
        [http://dx.doi.org/10.1016/j.ijcard.2009.09.436]

[8]   Modi J, Sharma P, Earl A, Simpson M, Mitchell JR, Goyal M. iPhone-based teleradiology for the diagnosis of acute cervico-dorsal spine trauma. Can J Neurol Sci 2010; 37(6): 849-54.
        [http://dx.doi.org/10.1017/S0317167100051556] [PMID: 21059550]

[9]   Choudhri A F, Radvany M G. Initial Experience with a Handheld Device Digital Imaging and Communications in Medicine Viewer: OsiriX Mobile on the iPhone. J Digit Imaging 2010; 24-2: 184-9.

[10]   Arad E, Trinidad T. Are mobile phone-camera transmitted uro-radiograph images reliable in accurate diagnosis and prompt treatment of emergency urological conditions? J Endourol 2006; A285-5.

[11]   LaBounty TM, Kim RJ, Lin FY, Budoff MJ, Weinsaft JW, Min JK. Diagnostic accuracy of coronary computed tomography angiography as interpreted on a mobile handheld phone device. JACC Cardiovasc Imaging 2010; 3(5): 482-90.
        [http://dx.doi.org/10.1016/j.jcmg.2009.11.018] [PMID: 20466343]

[12]   Saha A, Liang H, *et al.* Assessment of Mobile Technologies for Displaying Medical Images. J Disp Technol 2008; 415-23.
        [http://dx.doi.org/10.1109/JDT.2008.924157]

[13]   Tang FH, Ng DKS, Chow DHK. An Image Feature Approach for Computer-aided Detection of Ischemic Stroke. Computers in Biology and Medicine 2011; 41(2011): 525-36.
        [http://dx.doi.org/10.1016/j.compbiomed.2011.05.001]

[14]   4G: https://en.wikipedia.org/wiki/4G access on 22 Jan 2017.

CHAPTER 3

Data Mining and Big Data in Medical Imaging

Abstract: The medical images in the Picture Archiving and Communication System (PACS) provide a resource for data mining and knowledge discovery. The information in the DICOM header can be extracted to produce meaningful information. We illustrate with two examples in the practice of medical imaging.

Keywords: Big data, Data mining, Dose monitoring, DICM, Medical imaging.

1. DATA MINING AND BIG DATA

Due to the technological advancement, the use of computer and the storage of data become a social phenomenon [1 - 4]. Be it in industries, the businesses, and science or medical fields, the use of electronic database is very common [1, 2], which pave the way to not only huge amount of storage, but data processing and calculation as well [3]. When there is a larger amount of data, there could be some underlying relationships and hidden patterns found among different variables [5, 6].

As these hidden associations are not easy to be discovered by human eye, data mining methods are created with a view to analyze the large amount of data and discover those hidden relationships by the computerized method. The meaning of data mining is to use computerized method to figure out additional information from a great amount of data [2 - 7]. Data mining is a complicated process making use of computer science, engineering and statistics [3, 6, 7]. Variables in a database can be analyzed by data mining methods to figure out useful information which can be applied in the reality to have better management of resources.

Data mining has been used in the field of radiography. The feasibility on improvement in radiography has been proven by several studies. Here are some examples: Ko *et al.* [8] proposed a data mining model to categorize plain X-ray images automatically and proved its success of the improvement in performance of classification performance and processing time. Other than image categorization, data mining is also able to extract useful information from medical images automatically for making diagnosis. This were proven by the research done by Linder *et al.* [9] and Cuingnet *et al.* [10], where data mining was applied in the segmentation of proximal femur in plain X-ray and segmentation of kidney in CT. Promising results were obtained in the above studies, which facilitate diagnosis of diseases. Many studies did statistics and calculation on the radiation dose or exposure index by the aid of data mining with the aim to improve radiography practice [11 - 13]. Yet, up till now, no studies have been reported involving analysis of factors or variables other than dosimetric data using data mining methods.

2. MEDICAL IMAGING AND DATA MINING

Imaging is more than pictures. They are part of big data analytics. Conventional imaging reading by radiologists can only uncover abnormalities and extent of pathology if disease is already diagnosed. Big data analytics, on the other hand can give personalized recommendations for precision personal care.

One potential is to quantify metrics of images according to image pixel analysis. Patient having dense breast tissue are already known to increase the risk of getting breast cancer [14, 15]. In order to aid the radiologist to accurately quantify breast density, new volumetric computer-aided thresholding algorithm like Volpara™ was developed to analyse the big data from image pixels of the digital mammograms. Accuracy was proved to be comparable to visual assessment [16], yet more efficient, objective and fully automated. Another example of utilizing big data analytics for image big data is the computation of coronary artery calcification (CAC) scores. CAC can accurately predict 5 to 15-year all-cause mortality risk in asymptomatic patients [17, 18].

The above mentioned big data examples show how big data analytics can be applied to image data in radiology. The risk factors generated will become very important health indicators for asymptomatic patients. Radiological information when combined with other areas of medicine like Genomic Medicine [19] and Clinical Laboratory data, they can be the foundations of personalized precision medicine [20].

3. CLINICAL ENVIRONMENT OF RADIOGRAPHY

There are a great variety of modalities in a radiology department, such as plain X-ray, CT, ultrasound, magnetic resonance imaging and nuclear medicine. Digitization of image data is adapted in most modern radiology department. It fosters giant databases containing both the medical images and their descriptive texts or numerical data [21, 22]. There is countless data recorded in these modalities, in which the database can reflect the clinical practice. These would be very valuable for analysis and can further be important indicators to improve the practice in radiography [21]. In the radiology field, PACS and DICOM can be the data sources for data mining. PACS is a computer network system in the medical field for data storage and transmission [21]. DICOM is the standard used in medical imaging all over the world, which enables the storage and delivery of images [23, 24].

4. DICOM EXTRACTION

As image information is stored in the form of DICOM header, data can be extracted for analysis purpose [11 - 13]. The data includes patient information, examination details and dosimetric data (Fig. **1**). The DICOM header extraction can be done by specially-decided software. Usually, data will undergo three steps, namely data acquisition, data processing and data organization for further analyzed [13, 23, 24]. Jahnen *et al.* (2011) developed a program ("PerMoS") for DICOM extraction of CT data [23]. Another DICOM header extraction program Radimetrics™ Enterprise Platform (REP) (Bayer HealthCare, Germany) is a web-based and vendor-neutral platform to summarize the patient dosimetric data and examination details. The merits of Radimetrics [25] are that they can connect to PACS of any hospitals remotely to acquire the data stored in the DICOM header.

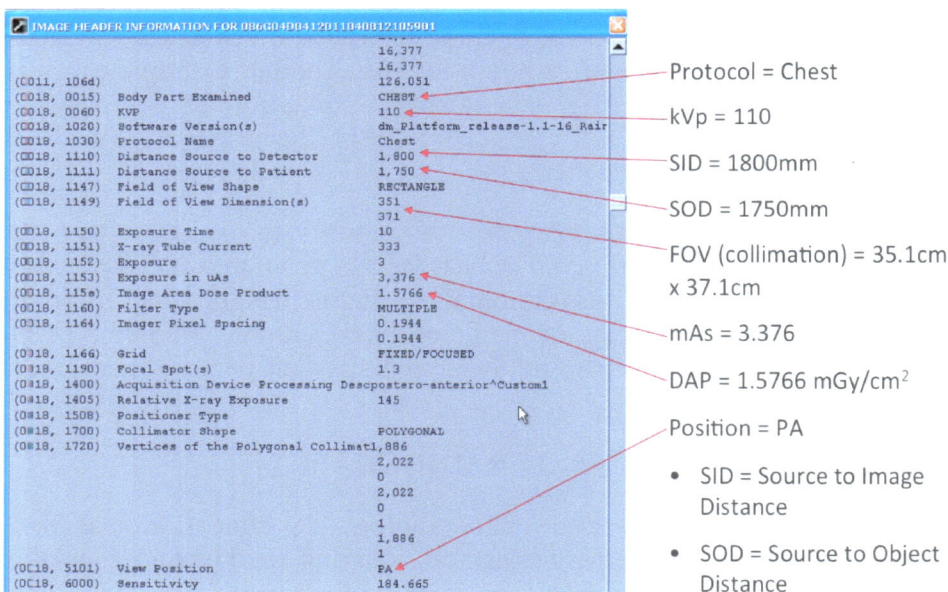

Fig. (1). DICOM Header of a DX image, with examination parameters and dose data shown.

As a radiation dose monitoring system, REP can extract relevant DICOM data from ionizing radiation producing modalities such as CT, PET/CT, NM, Mammo,

Fluoro, Angio, CR and DX. Extraction of DICOM data can done using Optical Character Recognition [26] from CT or Fluoro dose summary page as in Fig. (**2**) or direct extraction from DICOM header from CR, DX and Mammo. DICOM Modality Performed Procedure Step (MPPS) [27] and Radiation Dose Structure Report (RDSR) [28] are also supported. RDSR is developed as a DICOM standard for handling the recording and storage of radiation dose information from imaging modalities [29, 30] to replace legacy DICOM standard use for such purposes. Latest radiology devices like CT are always equipped with RDSR and are able to propagate dose data for estimation of radiation dose [28].

Patient Name:				Exam no: 1744	
Accession Number: ı				10 Aug 2009	
Patient ID:				Discovery CT750 HD	
Exam Description: CT HALS/THORAX/ABDOMEN					
		Dose Report			
Series	Type	Scan Range (mm)	CTDIvol (mGy)	DLP (mGy–cm)	Phantom cm
1	Scout	–	–	–	–
2	Helical	S15.750–I650.250	5.10	373.00	Body 32
5	Helical	S188.000–I105.000	5.10	182.72	Body 32
			Total Exam DLP:	555.72	
		1/1			

Fig. (2). Sample dose summary page from CT machine.

After dose information is fully acquired from examinations of the same protocol, dose report can be created. Dose standard such as Diagnostic Reference Level [31] can be generated using REP Dashboard functions and can be used as an optimization tool for dose reduction [32].

In addition, REP can do image pixel analytics (one kind of big data analytics) by obtaining the water equivalent diameter of the patients in different scan level. This can help to calculate the Size Specific Dose Estimates (see Fig. **3**), which is a more accurate patient dose calculation taking consideration for different sizes of patients [33, 34].

Many studies have used the dosimetric information in DICOM Header to help radiography practice for data mining [23, 24, 35, 36]. In our study, not only DICOM extraction of dosimetric data, but also other data in DICOM header such as patient information and examination details were used for data mining. The hidden relationship between different variables in DICOM header was explored.

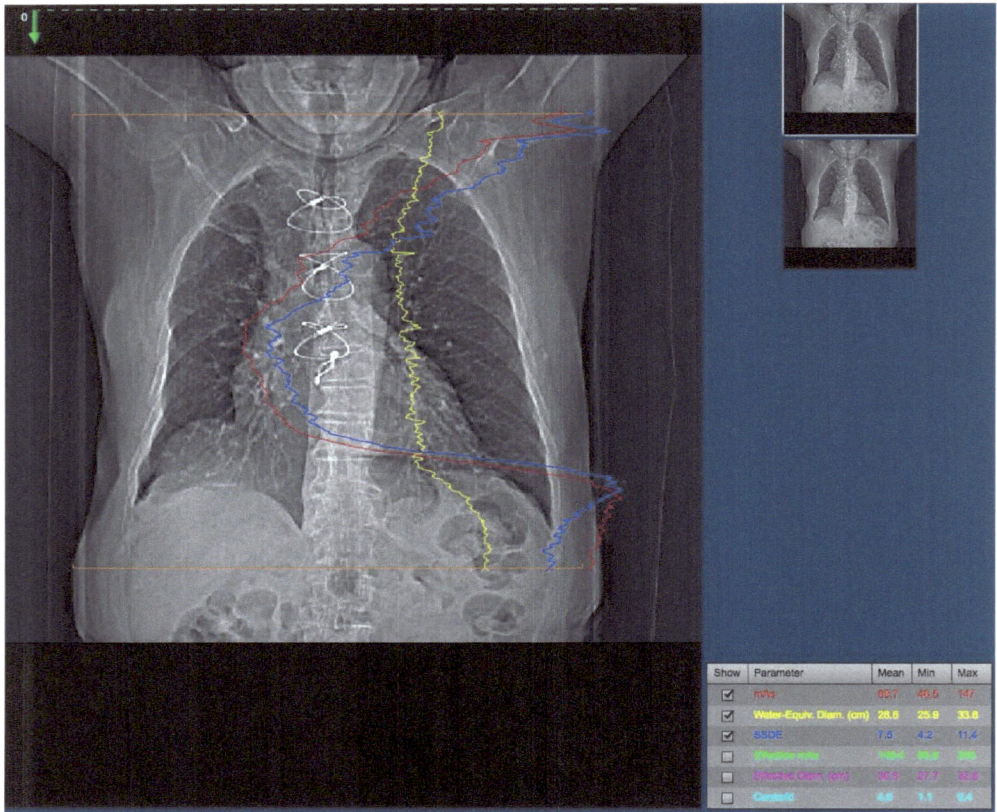

Fig. (3). Big data analytics to calculate Size Specific Dose Estimates (SSDE) using Water Equivalent Diameter (WED) in Radimetrics. Line in RED is mAs; Line in YELLOW is Water Equivalent Diameter; Line in BLUE is calculated SSDE using WED and mAs.

5. DATA PROCESSING SOFTWARE: R AND RATTLE

R is an open source software used for statistical computing and also a computing language [37]. It was developed in Bell Laboratories by John Chamber, making use of S programming language [38]. Heaps of statistics literatures have relationship with R [38 - 40] which means R is of good research value.

Rattle (R Analytical Tool to Learn Easily) is a free package in R designed for new users of data mining [41, 42] and therefore, provides simplified data mining process by a graphical user interface. Rattle paves a way to sophisticated tasks in R [41, 42] and provides different data mining tools, for example, clustering, decision tree and random forest. Rattle also provides statistical analysis tool for data mining such as the ROC curve study [42].

6. RANDOM FOREST

Random Forest is an ensemble data mining model of multiple decision trees for classification and regression which means the decision making by random forest involves multiple decision trees to vote [41].

A main feature of random forest is the randomness. Multiple trees are generated by the randomly selected sample and input attribute (input variable) [41, 43]. The randomness is one of the advantage of random forest to have greater robust to noisy data [41]. Since many trees are used in the decision, it can be regarded as testing the data with many models at the same time. This increases the accuracy of decision making of random forest and avoid overfitting which is a major problem in a single decision tree [41].

Apart from building decision-making models for data mining, random forest also allows users to measure the attribute importance [44]. The variable importance of the attributes can be measured quantitatively.

7. VARIABLE IMPORTANCE MEASURES

During the process of data in the random forest, several attributes with significance were picked up. The significance is called variable importance. Variable importance can be used as measurement in variable selection [44]. The higher the variable importance is, the more that input attribute affects the target. The random forest function in Rattle can generate two values to measure the variable importance, namely, mean decrease accuracy (MDA) and mean decrease Gini (MDG). Both MDA and MDG were used in predictor (attribute) selection in a lot of recent studies [44, 45].

MDA of a predictor is the normalized average of the difference among all trees between the accuracy (observations correctly classified) of a predictor and the accuracy after permuting this randomly selected predictor [44, 46]. The higher MDA is, the more important the predictor will be [47]. MDA has strong correlation for the top-ranked predictor [48] and therefore it can fit our study, which was to find out the most related attributes. MDG is the normalized average of decrease among all trees in node impurities from splitting a predictor [44, 46] The node impurity is measured by Gini coefficient which is a measurement of homogeneity of the nodes and leaves from 0 to 1, where 1 is the most heterogeneous [47]. The higher the MDG is, the higher purity of the node will be. The bias of MDG and MDA has been compared. It was suggested in some studies that the bias in MDG is the higher [44, 49]. Therefore, MDA was more preferred

8. USE OF DATA MINING IN DOSE MONITORING

We have conducted a study where the DICOM header of 3290 CT cases were extracted retrospectively from six clinical centers or hospitals in North America. It is possible to find hidden pattern in dataset less than 100 samples though it is relatively difficult. In the study conducted by Pechenizkiy *et al.*, 73 cases of online exams were used for data mining to determine hidden relationship in answering questions [15]. In the study conducted by Robin Genuer, only 72 cases of MRI were used for data mining of 1000 attributes to predict a behavioral variable based on random forest model [16]. In view of the possibility of determining patterns with dataset not more than 100 samples, the use of 3290 samples in our study is sufficient for data mining of 44 attributes based on the random forest model.

In our study, the meta-data hidden in the DICOM headers stored in the PACS was extracted by Radimetrics™ Enterprise Platform. Various parameters of the CT examinations include gender, age, height, weight, exposure parameters and doses of various body regions were acquired.

These samples were extracted in the form of .csv file and sent by the senior radiographers after the anonymization of patient information. Authorization from the Ethics Commission will be requested such that the confidentiality of collected data will be secured.

8.1. Whole Body Dose and Gender

The MDA of Gender is 15.12 when whole body dose was set as the target. These values were large when compared with other attributes (Fig. **4**). It indicates that there is a tendency for the attribute "Gender" having a stronger association with the whole body dose. Thus, gender was selected for further investigation of the association with whole body dose.

The associated Area Under the Curve (AUC) of whole body dose was 0.9966. which indicates that the built prediction model by random forest can make an accurate prediction during the application of model in the remaining 30 percent data. It implies that the prediction is likely to be accurate when this built prediction model applies to new-collected data.

Our result indicated that there was an association between gender and whole body dose (Chi-Square test, $p<0.05$), giving the mean of whole body dose male (0.729J) was significantly higher than that of female (0.657J) (Mann-Whitney U, $p<0.05$.

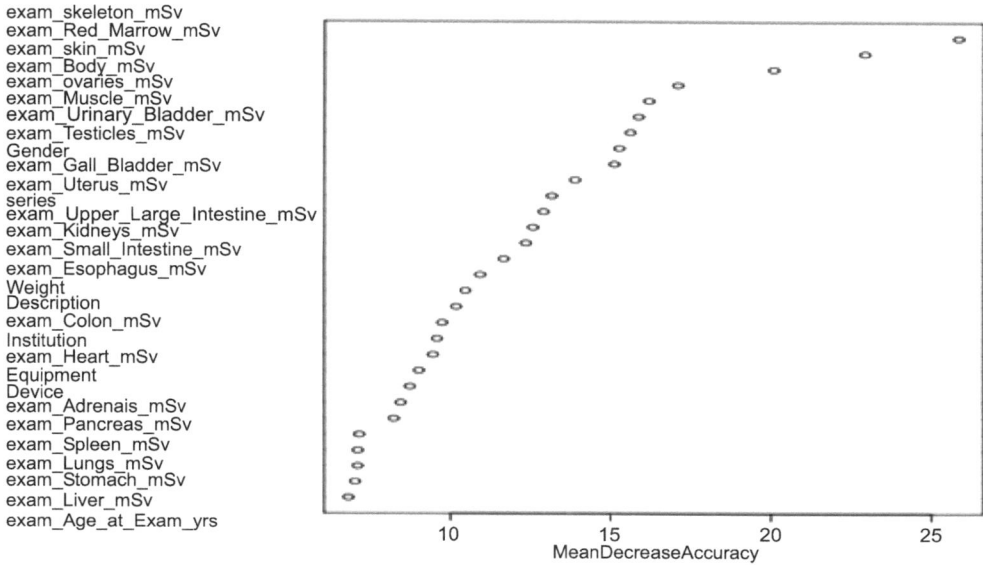

Fig. (4). Variable Importance of different attributes against MDA (Whole Body Dose as target).

Our finding indicates that the gender was associated to the whole body dose and the whole body dose received by male were greater than that by female. The direct study of relationship between gender and whole body dose was not noted in other study.

We do not stipulate any possible reasons for this phenomenon at this stage, but the data mining for medical imaging does discover associations of different factors that we may not be aware of.

9. DISCUSSION AND CONCLUSION

Data Mining and Big Data are two non-separable areas in Medical Imaging. Advances in computation means Big Data can be processed in real time to give immediate feedback. The calculation will be meaningful only if Data Mining methods developed can extract relevant relationship or metrics during the analytics. They can help to identify malignancies or predict abnormalities in Preventive Medicine. They can help to quantify the pathology and lead to effective treatment and better prognosis. They can also help to generate add-on benefits like machine utilization, staff performance, protocol management *etc*, that achieve quality assurance purposes.

However, finding relationships in vast amount of data is not an easy task. Particularly when imaging data are unstructured and extremely diverse in type and content. Building standards may be one way to ease data mining. For example using Report templates and standard wordings [50] can analysis more findings in radiology reports. Another solution is to build Artificial Intelligence for data mining from big data. Watson Project is building Cognitive systems that can understand, reason and learn. They will help people to expand their knowledge base, improve their productivity and deepen their expertise. Hidden health data are now visible [51]. Finally we need a really huge database for testing every new algorithm, data mining method or cognitive system. In America, we have different database like NLST [52], DMIST [53], and PLCO 56 that we can make use of for clinical trials. Commercial company like Zebra Medical Vision is building a mega database (10 million deidentified imaging studies in 2015) of medical imaging examinations [54] for this function.

CONFLICT OF INTEREST

The author(s) confirm that this chapter contents have no conflict of interest.

ACKNOWLEDGEMENTS

We thank Bayer Health Care for donation of the user license of Radimetrics™ Enterprise Platform (REP) for trial in this study.

REFERENCES

[1]   Han J, Kamber M. ScienceDirect (Online service), et al. Data mining concepts and techniques. 3rd ed., 2012. Waltham, Mass: Burlington, MA: Elsevier, c2012

[2]   Osmar Z. Principles of Knowledge Discovery in Databases 1999.

[3]   Suh S. Practical applications of data mining. Jones & Bartlett Publishers 2012.

[4]   Giudici P, Figini S. Applied data mining for business and industry. 2nd ed., John Wiley & Sons Ltd 2009.
      [http://dx.doi.org/10.1002/9780470745830]

[5]   Tan P, Steinbach M, Kumar V. Introduction to data mining. Pearson Addison Wesley Boston 2006.

[6]   Gorunescu F. Data mining concepts, models and techniques 2011.

[7]   Zhao Y. R and data mining: Examples and case studies. Academic Press 2012.

[8]   Ko BC, Kim SH, Nam JY. X-ray image classification using random forests with local wavelet-based CS-local binary patterns. J Digit Imaging 2011; 24(6): 1141-51.
      [http://dx.doi.org/10.1007/s10278-011-9380-3] [PMID: 21487837]

[9]   Lindner C, Thiagarajah S, Wilkinson JM, Wallis GA, Cootes TF, Cootes T. Fully automatic segmentation of the proximal femur using random forest regression voting. IEEE Trans Med Imaging 2013; 32(8): 1462-72.
      [http://dx.doi.org/10.1109/TMI.2013.2258030] [PMID: 23591481]

[10] Cuingnet R, Prevost R, Lesage D, Cohen LD, Mory B, Ardon R. Automatic detection and segmentation of kidneys in 3D CT images using random forests.Anonymous Medical Image Computing and Computer-Assisted Intervention–MICCAI 2012. Springer 2012; pp. 66-74.
      [http://dx.doi.org/10.1007/978-3-642-33454-2_9]

[11]   Rampado O, Garelli E, Zatteri R, Escoffier U, De Lucchi R, Ropolo R. Patient dose evaluation by means of DICOM images for a direct radiography system. Radiol Med (Torino) 2008; 113(8): 1219-28.
[http://dx.doi.org/10.1007/s11547-008-0339-5] [PMID: 18956145]

[12]   Stewart BK, Kanal KM, Perdue JR, Mann FA. Computed radiography dose data mining and surveillance as an ongoing quality assurance improvement process. AJR Am J Roentgenol 2007; 189(1): 7-11.
[http://dx.doi.org/10.2214/AJR.06.1232] [PMID: 17579143]

[13]   Vano E, Fernandez JM, Ten JI, Gonzalez L, Guibelalde E, Prieto C. Patient dosimetry and image quality in digital radiology from online audit of the X-ray system. Radiat Prot Dosimetry 2005; 117(1-3): 199-203.
[http://dx.doi.org/10.1093/rpd/nci716] [PMID: 16461529]

[14]   Ikuta I, Sodickson A, Wasser EJ, Warden GI, Gerbaudo VH, Khorasani R. Exposing exposure: enhancing patient safety through automated data mining of nuclear medicine reports for quality assurance and organ dose monitoring. Radiology 2012; 264(2): 406-13.
[http://dx.doi.org/10.1148/radiol.12111823] [PMID: 22627599]

[15]   Mykola P, Toon C, Ekaterina V, *et al.* Mining the Student Assessment Data: Lessons Drawn from a Small Scale Case Study. EDM 2008; pp. 187-91.

[16]   Robin G, Vincent M, Evelyn E, *et al.* Random Forests Based Feature Selection for Decoding fMRI Data. Proceedings Compstat 2010; 267: 1-8.

[17]   Fayyad U, Piatetsky-Shapiro G, Smyth P. From data mining to knowledge discovery in databases. AI Mag 1996; 17: 37.

[18]   Ramos-Pollán R, Guevara-López MÁ, Oliveira E. Introducing ROC curves as error measure functions: a new approach to train ANN-based biomedical data classifiers.Anonymous Progress in Pattern Recognition, Image Analysis, Computer Vision, and Applications Springer Berlin Heidelberg,. 2010; pp. 517-24.
[http://dx.doi.org/10.1007/978-3-642-16687-7_68]

[19]   Fawcett T. An introduction to ROC analysis. Pattern Recognit Lett 2006; 27: 861-74.
[http://dx.doi.org/10.1016/j.patrec.2005.10.010]

[20]   Utts J, Heckard R. Statistical ideas and methods. Cengage Learning 2005.

[21]   Kharat AT, Singh A, Kulkarni VM, Shah D. Data mining in radiology 2014.
[http://dx.doi.org/10.4103/0971-3026.134367]

[22]   Richard Chen M. Radiology Data Mining Applications using Imaging Informatics. InTech 2008.

[23]   Jahnen A, Kohler S, Hermen J, Tack D, Back C. Automatic computed tomography patient dose calculation using DICOM header metadata. Radiat Prot Dosimetry 2011; 147(1-2): 317-20.
[http://dx.doi.org/10.1093/rpd/ncr338] [PMID: 21831868]

[24]   Wang S, Pavlicek W, Roberts CC, *et al.* An automated DICOM database capable of arbitrary data mining (including radiation dose indicators) for quality monitoring. J Digit Imaging 2011; 24(2): 223-33.
[http://dx.doi.org/10.1007/s10278-010-9329-y] [PMID: 20824303]

[25]   The consistent quality of connected radiology , [Accessed 2 May 2016]; https://www.radio logysolutions.bayer.com/static/media/PDFs/2-1-2-1_Radimetrics_Enterprise_Platform/REP_ SeamslesslySmart.pdf

[26]   Optical character recognition , [Accessed 2 May 2016]; https://en.wikipedia.org/wiki/Optical_ character_recognition

[27]   DICOM standard supplement 17: Modality Performed Procedure Step. Rosslyn, Virginia: DICOM Standards Committee 1998.

[28] [Accessed 2 May 2016]; http://dicom.nema.org/documents/ CT_Dose_Information_in_DICOM_Data-DICOM_FAQ.pdf

[29] DICOM standard supplement 127: CT radiation dose reporting. Rosslyn, Virginia: DICOM Standards Committee 2007.

[30] DICOM standard part 16: content mapping resource. Rosslyn, Virginia: DICOM Standards Committee 2008.

[31] [Accessed 2 May 2016]; https://rpop.iaea.org/RPOP/RPoP/Content/InformationFor/HealthProfessionals/1_Radiology/ComputedTomography/diagnostic-reference-levels.htm

[32] Diagnostic Reference Levels in Medical Imaging: Review and additional advice. ICRP Committee 3 2001.

[33] Size-Specific Dose Estimates (SSDE) in Pediatric and Adult Body CT Examinations. AAPM Task Group 204 2011.

[34] Use of Water Equivalent Diameter for Calculating Patient Size and Size-Specific Dose Estimates (SSDE) in CT. AAPM Task Group 220 2014.

[35] Cohen MD, Markowitz R, Hill J, Huda W, Babyn P, Apgar B. Quality assurance: a comparison study of radiographic exposure for neonatal chest radiographs at 4 academic hospitals. Pediatr Radiol 2012; 42(6): 668-73.
[http://dx.doi.org/10.1007/s00247-011-2290-1] [PMID: 22057362]

[36] Källman HE, Halsius E, Folkesson M, Larsson Y, Stenström M, Båth M. Automated detection of changes in patient exposure in digital projection radiography using exposure index from DICOM header metadata. Acta Oncol 2011; 50(6): 960-5.
[http://dx.doi.org/10.3109/0284186X.2011.579622] [PMID: 21767197]

[37] Fox J, Andersen R. Using the R statistical computing environment to teach social statistics courses. Department of Sociology, McMaster University 2005.

[38] Chambers JM. Programming with data: A guide to the S language. Springer Science & Business Media 1998.
[http://dx.doi.org/10.1007/978-1-4684-6306-4]

[39] Pinheiro JC, Bates DM. Mixed-effects models in S and S-PLUS. Springer Science & Business Media 2000.
[http://dx.doi.org/10.1007/978-1-4419-0318-1]

[40] Venables WN, Ripley BD. Modern applied statistics with S. Springer Science & Business Media 2002.
[http://dx.doi.org/10.1007/978-0-387-21706-2]

[41] Williams GJ. Data Mining with Rattle and R: The Art of Excavating Data for Knowledge Discovery. Springer Science & Business Media 2011; p. 374.
[http://dx.doi.org/10.1007/978-1-4419-9890-3]

[42] Williams GJ. Rattle: A data mining GUI for R. R J 2009; 1: 45-55.

[43] Mitchell TM. Machine learning 1997. Burr Ridge, IL: McGraw Hill 1997; p. 45.

[44] Strobl C, Boulesteix AL, Zeileis A, Hothorn T. Bias in random forest variable importance measures: illustrations, sources and a solution. BMC Bioinformatics 2007; 8: 25.
[http://dx.doi.org/10.1186/1471-2105-8-25] [PMID: 17254353]

[45] Louppe G, Wehenkel L, Sutera A, Geurts P. Understanding variable importances in forests of randomized trees. Adv Neural Inf Process Syst 2013; 431-9.

[46] Nicodemus KK. Letter to the editor: on the stability and ranking of predictors from random forest variable importance measures. Brief Bioinform. 2011; 12: pp. 369-73.

[47] Liaw A, Wiener M. Classification and regression by randomForest. R News 2002; 2: 18-22.

[48] Breiman L. Random forests. Mach Learn 2001; 45: 5-32.
[http://dx.doi.org/10.1023/A:1010933404324]

[49] White AP, Liu WZ. Technical note: Bias in information-based measures in decision tree induction. Mach Learn 1994; 15: 321-9.
[http://dx.doi.org/10.1007/BF00993349]

[50] RadLex in Your Practice , [Accessed 14 June 2016]; https://www.rsna.org/RadLex_in_Your_Practice.aspx

[51] Watson Health BM. [Accessed 14 June 2016]; http://www.ibm.com/smarterplanet/us/en/ibmwatson/health/

[52] [Accessed 14 June 2016]; http://www.cancer.gov/types/lung/research/nlst

[53] [Accessed 14 June 2016]; http://www.acr.org/About-Us/Media-Center/ Position-Statements/Positio-Statements-Folder/ACR-Statement-Regarding-the-Digital-Mammographic-Imaging-Screeing-Trial-DMIST-Results

[54] Vision ZM. Imaging Analytics We are teaching computers to detect and diagnose critical medical conditions , [Accessed 14 June 2016]; https://www.zebra-med.com/imaging-analytics/

PART II: MEDICAL IMAGING FOR BETTER HEALTH AND DISEASE DETECTION

CHAPTER 4

Computer Aided Detection in Medical Imaging

Abstract: Computer aided diagnosis or detection is a computer system to assist medical doctors to improve the accuracy and efficiency of health care. We describe a computer-aided detection method for stroke as an example to illustrate the steps describing this method.

Keywords: Computer-aided detection, Computer-aided diagnosis, Stroke.

1. INTRODUCTION

Computer aided diagnosis CADx or detection (CADe), sometimes refers as CAD, is the system that aims to assist medical personnel in the image interpretation by computer outputs of the predictive value of medical images. Specialists, as human, can make errors during interpretation due to fatigue, overload of information, and variable environmental conditions. On the other hand, with the advent of multi-detector CT, there is an increasing volume of imaging data. The use of CAD system provides a more efficient means of processing image data and it offers a "second opinion" to assist doctors' clinical decision.

Essentially CAD consists of the following steps:

1. Image acquisition: Images are digitized or acquired from imaging modalities. With the PACS in place, images can be directly transfer to the CAD workstation.
2. Feature extraction: This includes image preprocessing and enhancement, segmentation. The noise and artefacts of images are reduced or removed. The regions of interest are segmented.
3. Quantitation of image features: ROI is translated to parameters that the CAD algorithms can processed.
4. Feature classification: This involves pattern recognition and artificial neural networks (ANNs). The ANNs can help to improve sensitivity and specificity of the CAD performance through feedback mechanisms.

5. Clinical decision and evaluation: Observer performance studies. This is usually the involvement of Receiver Operating Characteristics (ROC) study where specialists are recruited for evaluation of the images. On the other hand, numerical model observer plays an emerging role in assessing performance of the imaging system [25].

CAD has been applied in imaging modalities such as plain radiography, CT, MRI, etc. in areas such as the detection of breast lesions on mammograms [1], lung nodules in chest [2] and CT lung [3], and polyps in CT colonography [4]. It also helps in thyroid nodule detection [5], finding cell nuclei [6] and midline tracing in brain CT [7].

2. CAD METHOD IN THE DETECTION OF STROKE

To illustrate the CAD method, here we used our developed CAD for stroke as an example.

2.1. Background of Study

The use of mathematical models for CAD has achieved certain success in the medical science. A study [8] shows that stroke is the result of the obstruction of one or more blood vessels to the brain and can be divided into hemorrhagic and ischemic strokes. Ischemic stroke is not obvious in imaging scan, as it appears as a small radiolucent area of less than 1.5cm in diameter on CT images [8]. Clinically, CT examination is preferred for patients with suspected stroke because it is readily accessible in general hospitals with relatively short examination time while the efficiency of examination is critical for patient survival and recovery [9].

Clinical diagnosis of ischemic stroke is difficult in the first three hours after the onset of stroke as the ischemic features are not apparent [10]. Study [11] showed that small lesion might not be detected with diffusion-weighted Magnetic Resonance Imaging (DWMRI). Therefore, a sensitive detection method that incorporates computer-aided detection method for stroke is critical and this demands more effective ways to improve detection rates.

Previous attempts have been made for the detection of acute stroke such as using a standard atlas of normalized CT images to identify hypodensity areas in the lentiform nucleus of the brain [12]; noise reduction by an adaptive partial smoothing filter (APSF) [13]; contrast enhancement by wavelet image processing [14]. Methods like wavelet decomposition of the histogram and energy difference measure are also attempts to detect delicate stroke changes [15]. However, their sample size was small and the detection is not fully automatic. It follows that an automatic CAD for stroke scheme required further elaboration and improvement.

The CAD stroke can be implemented in two stages.

Stage one is the establishment of an intelligent system for detection of stroke. This stage includes improvement of existing algorithm to detect and locate ischemic and hemorrhagic stroke. We adopted the Circular Adaptive Region of Interest (CAROI) method we proposed to detect subtle density change in ischemic stroke.

The CAROI method

The following briefly summarizes the CAROI method; the details are described in our earlier work [16]:

In this method, we generate a CAROI with radius, r = 5 pixels from one side of the brain. The CAROI grows with $r = 5,7,9....2n+1$. By comparing the total pixel value of CAROI $(i+1)$ with that of CAROI (i) iteratively, we are able to determine the subtle change in brain density (Fig. **1**). When a region of decrease is noted on one side of the brain, the correlation factor with the corresponding area on the other side of the brain is calculated.

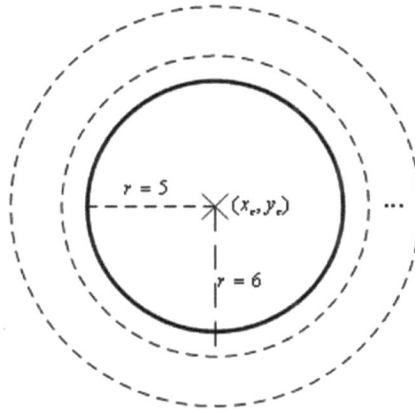

Fig. (1). The Circular Adaptive Regions of Interest.

The region of potential ischemic stroke can be located if the suspicious region has a low correlation factor with the corresponding region on the other side. Fig. (**2**) shows the suspicious region of density as located by CAROI. Once the region of suspected stroke is located, the image textual features such as correlation, standard deviation, energy, and entropy will be calculated. The calculated value of image textual feature will be used for training of the artificial neural network (ANN) method to rule out false positive and false negative regions. Fig. (**3**) is an example which demonstrates that stroke is detected at the caudate nucleus of right brain by CAD (Fig. **3b**).

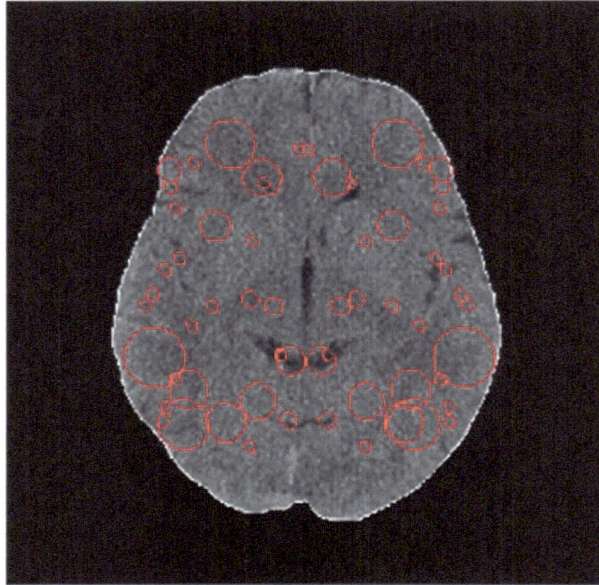

Fig. (2). The generated circular region of interests.

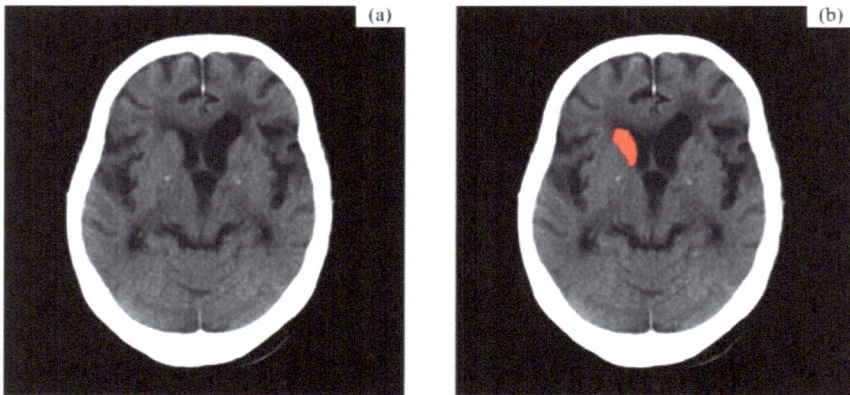

Fig. (3). (a) CT image before CAD, (b) Location of possible stroke by CAD.

For determination of hemorrhagic stroke, since there is usually an increase in radio-opacity, detection of area of stroke can be performed by thresholding method. For subtle increase in density, it can also be detected by CAROI method. However, in this case, the total pixel value of CAROI (i+1) should be greater than that of CAROI (i).

In order to establish the ANN model, CT brain images including 26 cases of stroke patients and 26 cases of non-stroke patients were collected from a local hospital retrospectively for training and testing of the model by round-robin (leave-one -out) method. This method is useful for limited sample collected for ANNs. All images were anonymized before leaving the PACS workstation.

Stage Two is the evaluation of outcomes. The performance of the system is evaluated in terms of users' performance for the CAD system.

2.3. Image Feature-Based Analysis

After the areas of stroke were detected automatically by the Stroke CAD program. The suspected region (if any) with a 20x20 pixel ROI was then extracted for image feature analysis. The extracted ROI was then used to compute the image feature parameters based on the gray level co-occurrence matrix.

In this study, 22 image features were used, which included: contrast, correlation, entropy, energy, homogeneity, autocorrelation, dissimilarity, information measure of correlation 1, information measure of correlation 2, sum average, sum variance, sum entropy, difference variance, difference entropy, sum of squares of variance, angular second moment, cluster shade, cluster prominence, maximum correlation coefficient, maximum probability, inverse difference normalized and inverse difference moment normalized [17, 18]. The numeric values of these image features from different approaches were then input for training and evaluating ANN classifiers.

2.5. ANNs Training and Testing

The numeric values of image feature parameters of 52 processed CT brain images (26 with stroke lesion and 26 without stroke lesion) were input for training ANN classifiers separately in the CAD system using leave-one-out method [19, 20]. By leave-one-out method, for each time, 51 images were used for training and one image was left out to test if the image was a stroke case or not until all 52 images were tested. The percentages of likelihood of stroke and non-stroke for each image were calculated.

2.6. Observer Test for The CAD System by Model Observer

2.6.1. Model Observer

Mathematical Model Observer models are designed to make decisions in detection tasks. Channelized Hotelling Observer (CHO) is one of the Model Observers that can pre-process the images with channel filters that are chosen to present the spatial frequency response of the human visual system. Previous studies have proven that CHO can be used to simulate as a human observer for assessment of classification tasks [21 - 24]. It is able to predict the human observer performance accurately and in a consistent manner for CT imaging and correlate well with human observers when proper channels were used. In this study, The Model Observer was used to read the 52 cases to simulate human observer to generate the Receiver Operating Curve (ROC) curve. This will be used to compare with the ROC study of the same cases detected by CAD with ANNs.

3. RESULTS

3.1. Performances of ANNs Classifiers

When ANNs were applied for these 52 images after training, the likelihood of stroke for each image was calculated. We defined the threshold that when the likelihood ≥50% that image presented a stroke feature, otherwise it was normal. The sensitivity, specificity and accuracy of ANNs classifier were 88.5%, 92.3% and 90.4% respectively

A ROC curve was generated for images using CAD system with ANN classifier in stroke detection. Another ROC curve was generated for images without CAD-ANN by Model observer that simulated reading by physicians (Fig. **4**). It was noted that for CAD-ANN, the area under the curve (Az) was 0.97 and that without CAD-ANN was 0.7149. There was a significant difference that using the CAD system with ANN classifier had could a significant improvement in detection of acute stroke ($p < 0.01$, chi-square test).

4. CONCLUDING REMARKS

It appears that the use of cloud computing can expand and extend CAD stroke system to the mobile technology as it allows a mobile device to perform computational demanding task of CAD by sharing the application of Stroke CAD in the cloud. The likelihood of stroke can return back to mobile devices to facilitate efficient use of CAD system.

We have used the CAD detection of stroke as an example to illustrate how is CAD realized in the clinical environment.

	Az-value	p-value
ANN	0.97	0.0058
MO-DICOM	0.7149	

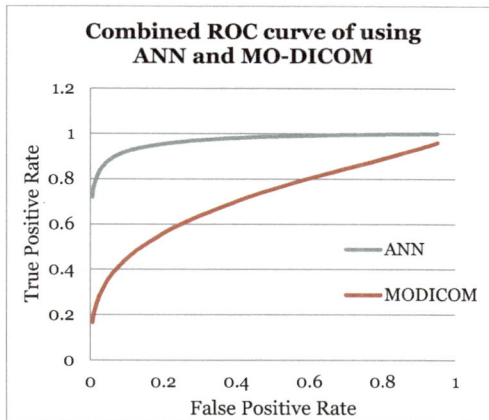

Fig. (4). Comparison of ROC curves of the CAD system with ANN classifier and Model Observer tested with the extracted DICOM sample images.

CONFLICT OF INTEREST

The author(s) confirm that this chapter contents have no conflict of interest.

ACKNOWLEDGEMENTS

Declared none

REFERENCES

[1]   Giger ML, Huo Z, Kupinski MA, Vyborny CJ. Computer aided diagnosis in mammography.Bellingham, WA: SPIE 2000; pp. 915-1004. The handbook of medical imaging, Vol. 2. Medical imaging processing and analysis.
      [http://dx.doi.org/10.1117/3.831079.ch15]

[2]   Xu XW, Doi K, Kobayashi T, MacMahon H, Giger ML. Development of an improved CAD scheme for automated detection of lung nodules in digital chest images. Med Phys 1997; 24(9): 1395-403.
      [http://dx.doi.org/10.1118/1.598028] [PMID: 9304567]

[3]   Jiang H, Yamamoto S, Iisaku S, *et al.* Computer-aided diagnosis system for lung cancer screening by CT.Computer-aided diagnosis in medical imaging. Amsterdam, The Neterlands: Elsevier 1999; pp. 125-30.

[4]   Jerebko AK, Malley JD, Franaszek M, Summers RM. Multiple neural network classification scheme for detection of colonic polyps in CT colonography data sets. Acad Radiol 2003; 10: 154-60.81. Na¨ppi J, Yoshida H. Feature-guided analysis.
      [http://dx.doi.org/10.1016/S1076-6332(03)80039-9]

[5]   Maroulis DE, Savelonas MA, Karkanis SA, Iakovidis DK, Dimitropoulos N. Computer-aided thyroid nodule detection in ultrasound images 18th IEEE Symposium on Computer-Based Medical Systems (CBMS'05). 271-6.
      [http://dx.doi.org/10.1109/CBMS.2005.44]

[6]   Byun J, Verardo MR, Sumengen B, Lewis GP, Manjunath BS, Fisher SK. Automated tool for the detection of cell nuclei in digital microscopic images: application to retinal images. Mol Vis 2006; 12: 949-60.

[PMID: 16943767]

[7]   Liao CC, Xiao F, Wong JM, Chiang IJ. A simple genetic algorithm for tracing the deformed midline on a single slice of brain CT using quadratic Bézier curves. 6th IEEE International Conference on Data Mining Workshops. 463-7.

[8]   de Haan RJ, Limburg M, Van der Meulen JH, Jacobs HM, Aaronson NK. Quality of life after stroke. Impact of stroke type and lesion location. Stroke 1995; 26(3): 402-8.
[http://dx.doi.org/10.1161/01.STR.26.3.402] [PMID: 7886714]

[9]   Adams H, Adams R, Del Zoppo G, Goldstein LB. Guidelines for the early management of patients with ischemic stroke: 2005 guidelines update a scientific statement from the Stroke Council of the American Heart Association/American Stroke Association. Stroke 2005; 36(4): 916-23.
[http://dx.doi.org/10.1161/01.STR.0000163257.66207.2d] [PMID: 15800252]

[10]   Toni D, Iweins F, von Kummer R, *et al.* Identification of lacunar infarcts before thrombolysis in the ECASS I study. Neurology 2000; 54(3): 684-8.
[http://dx.doi.org/10.1212/WNL.54.3.684] [PMID: 10680804]

[11]   Winbeck K, Bruckmaier K, Etgen T, von Einsiedel HG, Röttinger M, Sander D. Transient ischemic attack and stroke can be differentiated by analyzing early diffusion-weighted imaging signal intensity changes. Stroke 2004; 35(5): 1095-9.
[http://dx.doi.org/10.1161/01.STR.0000125720.02983.fe] [PMID: 15060321]

[12]   Talairach J, Tournoux P. A Co-Planar Stereotaxic Atlas of the Human Brain: An Approach to Medical Cerebral Imaging. New York: Thieme 1988.

[13]   Lee Y, Takahashi N, Tsai DY, Fujita H. Detectability improvement of early sign of acute stroke on brain CT images using an adaptive partial smoothing filter. Proc Soc Photo Opt Instrum Eng Med Imaging 2006; 6144: 2138-45.

[14]   Przelaskowski A, Sklinda K, Bargieł P, Walecki J, Biesiadko-Matuszewska M, Kazubek M. Improved early stroke detection: wavelet-based perception enhancement of computerized tomography exams. Comput Biol Med 2007; 37(4): 524-33.
[http://dx.doi.org/10.1016/j.compbiomed.2006.08.004] [PMID: 16999952]

[15]   Chawla M, Sharma S, Sivaswamy J, Kishore LT. A method for automatic detection and classification of stroke from brain CT images. Engineering in Medicine and Biology Society, 2009 EMBC 2009 Annual International Conference of the IEEE.
[http://dx.doi.org/10.1109/IEMBS.2009.5335289]

[16]   Tang FH, Ng DKS, Chow DHK. An Image Feature Approach for Computer-aided Detection of Ischemic Stroke. Computers in Biology and Medicine 2011; 41(2011): 525-36.
[http://dx.doi.org/10.1016/j.compbiomed.2011.05.001]

[17]   Haralick R, Shanmugam K, Dinstein I. Textural features for image classification. IEEE Trans Syst Man Cybern 1973; (6): 610-21.
[http://dx.doi.org/10.1109/TSMC.1973.4309314]

[18]   Ehsanirad A, Sharath Kumar Y. Leaf recognition for plant classification using GLCM and PCA methods. Oriental Journal of Computer Science and Technology 2010; 3(1): 31-6.

[19]   Wong T. Performance evaluation of classification algorithms by k-fold and leave-one-out cross validation. Pattern Recognit 2015; 1-8.

[20]   Leave-one-out demonstration [Internet]. [cited 14 April 2015]. Available from: https://www.projectrhea.org/rhea/images/3/39/Fig_Old_Kiwi.jpg

[21]   Gifford HC, King MA, de Vries DJ, Soares EJ. Channelized hotelling and human observer correlation for lesion detection in hepatic SPECT imaging. J Nucl Med 2000; 41(3): 514-21.
[PMID: 10716327]

[22]   Li K, Garrett J, Chen G. Correlation between human observer performance and model observer

performance in differential phase contrast CT. Medical Physics 2013; 40(11): 111905.1-.
[http://dx.doi.org/10.1118/1.4822576]

[23]   Leng S, Yu L, Zhang Y, *et al.* Correlation between model observer and human observer performance in CT imaging when lesion location is uncertain. Medical Physics 2013; 40(8): 081908.1-.
[http://dx.doi.org/10.1118/1.4812430]

[24]   Barrett HH, Yao J, Rolland JP, Myers KJ. Model observers for assessment of image quality. Proc Natl Acad Sci USA 1993; 90(21): 9758-65.
[http://dx.doi.org/10.1073/pnas.90.21.9758] [PMID: 8234311]

[25]   He Xin, Park Subok. Model Observers in Medical Imaging Research. Theranostics 2017; 3.10(2013): 774-86. PMC. Web. 7 Apr. 2017.

CHAPTER 5

Use of Biomechanical Engineering Method in Image Registration of Breast

Abstract:

Background: The image registration using positron emission tomography (PET) and magnetic resonance imaging (MRI) has been studied extensively. The purpose of this project is to propose a patient-specific image registration model that can improve both the accuracy and efficiency of the registration process. Large-scale deformation of the breast makes image registration of the breast a challenging task. Usually, a patient undergoes MRI in the prone position and PET in the supine position. Registration of breast in supine position with breast in prone position is a challenge.

Methods: Eight cases with corresponding pairs of PET/computed tomography (CT) and MRI breast images were used in this study for the performance of PET/MRI registration. Registration was based on a biomechanical finite element model that could simulate large-scale deformation of the breast under pressure.

Results: In this study, an accurate patient-specific registration model was built with a target registration error (TRE) of 4.77±2.20 mm.

Conclusion: Image deformation due to the effect of gravity was successfully modeled by the finite element method.

Keywords: Finite Element Analysis, Breast Modeling, PET and MR Registration.

1. INTRODUCTION

Breast cancer is considered as the second leading cause of cancer among females worldwide. According to cancer facts and figures published in 2016, the predicted number of new female breast cancer cases in the United States is 246,660 [1]. Better treatments can reduce mortality and change patients' life quality. The breast is a soft tissue that deforms very easily in different postures. Physical simulations for large deformations of the breast are crucial for many medical applications, such as image registration, image-guided surgery, cancer diagnosis and surgical planning [2]. Building a mechanical model is a promising contribution in the field of medical application.

Fuk-hay Tang

Finite element analysis (FEA) [3] is widely used in engineering areas, such as civil engineering and mechanical engineering. In this project, we used FEA to establish a registration model of breast images, particularly for breast MR and CT/PET images. As this process is highly correlated with material properties, registration integrated by FEA is more patient-specific.

Studies devoted to modeling the deformation of breast tissue have interested many researchers [4 - 12]. Biomechanical modeling has been used to simulate deformations of the breast under gravity loading [2, 6, 11], compression of mammography [7, 12], and biopsy processes [8]. However, none of these studies have used material properties as a patient-dependent parameter. A breast mainly consists of soft tissues, specifically, adipose and fibro-glandular tissues. A breast with more adipose is softer, and the deformation will be larger. This poses a challenging problem for researchers. Additionally, except for the difference in the density between adipose and fibro-glandular tissues, the distribution of fibro-glandular tissue, Cooper's line and skin also influence deformation. The proposed registration model based on finite element analysis will take the properties of these materials into consideration.

Different imaging modalities have been used for detecting breast cancer, such as CT, MRI, X-ray mammography and PET. PET is a molecular imaging modality that can recognize breast cancer at the molecular level to achieve early diagnosis and treatment. To enhance the image quality of PET, a registration process to fuse PET images with MRI that contains anatomical structural information is necessary [13]. Due to the differences in the resolution of PET and MRI scans and the image formation processes, the intensity relationship of PET and MR images cannot be defined. The registration of MR and PET scans based on similarity measures provides unsatisfactory results [14]. The accurate three-dimensional registration of PET and MR images of the breast can provide additional valuable information by combining functional information with anatomical information [15]. Here, we propose an FEA-based registration model for PET and MRI scans, which takes patient-specific features into consideration.

2. METHODOLOGY

The whole registration process follows the flowchart in Fig. (**1**). In this project, the MRI images were the target images and the PET/CT images were the float images. The three-dimensional (3D) model was built based on CT images to keep the internal structural information. As PET and CT scans share the same coordinate system, registrations were directly applied to the CT and MRI images and then the deformation was translated to PET images. Firstly, the CT images were segmented and cropped to generate a 3D breast model. Secondly, finite element analysis was performed on the 3D model to predict breast deformation. Thirdly, the FEA results were exported to generate deformed CT images, the deformed CT images were registered with MR images by affine transformation, and the transformations were applied to PET images to finish the PET/MRI registration.

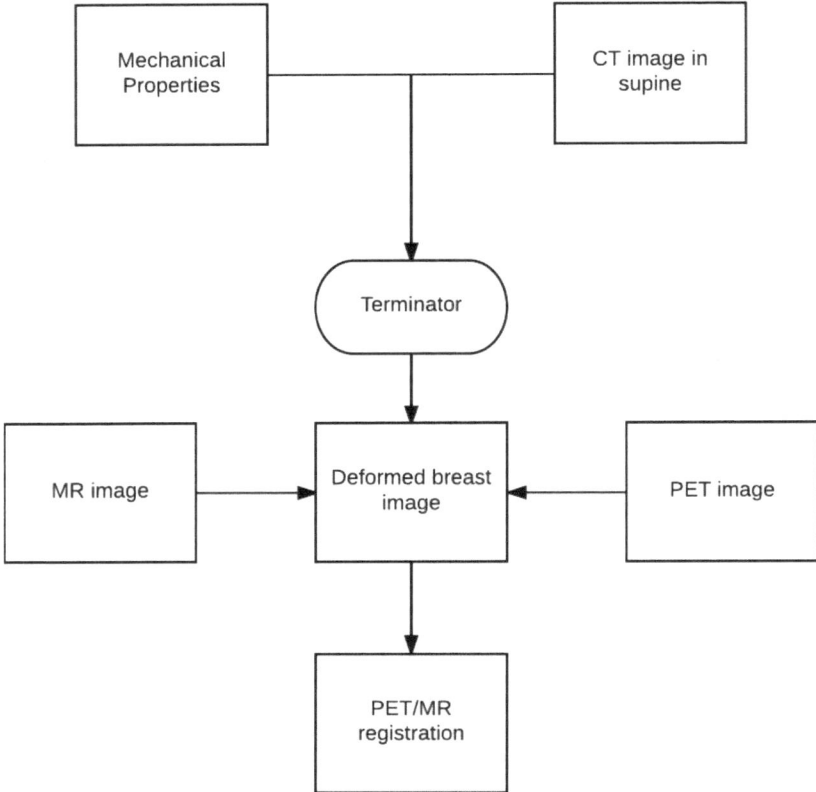

Fig. (1). The registration flowchart.

2.1. Preprocessing

Eight cases of corresponding pairs of MR images and PET/CT images collected from a local private hospital were used in this study. In each case, the CT images were cropped, and the left or right breast was selected based on the lesion on MR images. Breast images between the second and the seventh ribs were used to build a breast model. Cooper's ligaments were ignored because they were not visible in these images. The CT breast images were segmented into adipose and fibro-glandular tissues automatically using the fuzzy C-means algorithm [16]. The chest wall and muscle were segmented manually from the breast, and then the 3D model of fat tissue and fibro-glandular tissue (Fig. **2**) was built based on these segmented images *via* a marching cube operation [17].

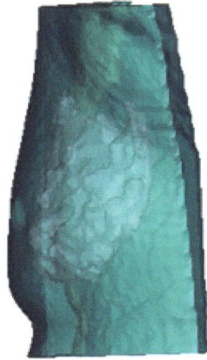

Fig. (2). Segmented breast model. (Fat tissue is in the green color, and fibro-glandular tissue is in the light gray color).

2.2. The Patient-Specific Model

As shown in Fig. (**2**), a three-dimensional breast model was generated by merging the fat model (green color) and the fibro-glandular model (light gray color) together. The finite element method (FEM) was used to simulate the physical behavior of the breast during the deformation process.

In order to improve the efficiency of operation during finite element analysis, the model was cut into cubes to generate finer hexahedron meshes as shown in Fig. (**3a**) and (**3b**). The model was assigned with a homogeneous isotropic material. The stiffness ratio between fibro-glandular tissue and fatty tissue was chosen based on the published data; the Young's modulus of fibro-glandular tissue is modeled 7.5 higher than that of fatty tissue [18]. The Poisson ratio used in this study was 0.45 because the breast was considered to be incompressible according to previous studies [4, 6, 19, 20]. A Neo-Hookean constitutive relationship was used to predict the nonlinear stress-strain behavior of hyperplastic materials [21] and has been proven to reliably and accurately represent the mechanical behavior of incompressible isotropic soft tissue [22, 23]. The physical behavior was also described by boundary conditions, in which the surface connected to the chest wall was fixed in an anterior-posterior direction to simulate the fixation at the chest wall [18].

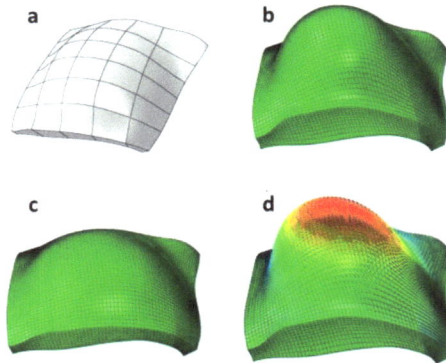

Fig. (3). a, a 3D breast model was generated, and to create a finer mesh, the 3D model was segmented into small cubes. **b**, hexahedron meshes were created based on cubes. **c**, after the defining loading, the boundary condition and mechanical properties, breast deformation under gravity was simulated. **d**, the nodal deformation vector was plotted on each node to illustrate how the node moves during deformation.

2.3. Deformation Simulation

The breast deformation was predicted using ABAQUS [24]. Displacements equal to zero were assigned to the surface connected to the chest wall in X, Y, and Z directions. Gravity loading was added along the vertical direction.

All images (CT, PET and MRI) of the breast were obtained under a gravity loading environment. Therefore, the model built from these images is a deformed model in the loading condition. The identification of the reference state (load-free state) of the breast is required, which can make the prediction of deformation more reliable [25]. Rajagopal *et al*. [20] developed a method to calculate the reference state of the breast by an iterative process. However, this method was very complicated. A simple way to find the reference state is to calculate the internal stress of the breast in supine position and then to release it.

The initial material properties of the breast for input are shown in Table **1**. The deformed model after FEA is shown in Fig. (**3c**).

Table 1. Initial material properties of the breast.

	Density (kg/m3)	Young's Modulus (kPa)	Poisson Ratio
Fat	1000	250	0.45
Fibro-glandular	1200	1875	0.45

The affine transformation was combined with FEA deformable registration in this project to formalize a hybrid registration, which can further improve the registration quality. As CT and PET share the same coordinate system, the affine transformation was conducted on a CT image and then transferred to a PET image.

3. RESULTS

Eight sets of breast images were collected in this project. For each image set, the patient had undergone CT/PET and MR examinations. The case information of these images is shown in Table **2**.

Table 2. Breast image basic information: volume and density of the breast image, the age of the patient, the lesion diameter, and the fibro-glandular tissue diameter.

Case no.	Volume (ml)	Age (years)	Lesion Diameter (mm)	Fibro-glandular Diameter (mm)	Density
S1	386	41	37	37	0.46
S2	1072	46	14.8	68	0.17
S3	852	77	23.8	106	0.13
S4	776	63	18.3	143	0.27
S5	766	33	4.6	167	0.13
S6	582	27	30.1	60	0.57
S7	670	39	22.5	185	0.36
S8	757	34	61.3	103	0.46

Fig. (**4**) presents the registered PET/MR image, with the lesion in the PET image marked as red. The registered PET/MR image of Case No.5 was not shown in Fig. (**4**) because there is no clear lesion in the image. Our method accurately predicted the location of the lesion with a TRE=4.77±2.20 mm.

4. DISCUSSION

4.1. Modeling Process

In this paper, we presented a hybrid approach for the registration of MR images in the prone position and PET/CT images in the supine position. Firstly, the large deformation was simulated by a finite element method, which was a 3D/3D surface-based registration. Secondly, an affine transformation was applied to the FEA of the deformed image to finish further hybrid registration. The hybrid registration method can improve the accuracy of purely FEA deformed registration [26].

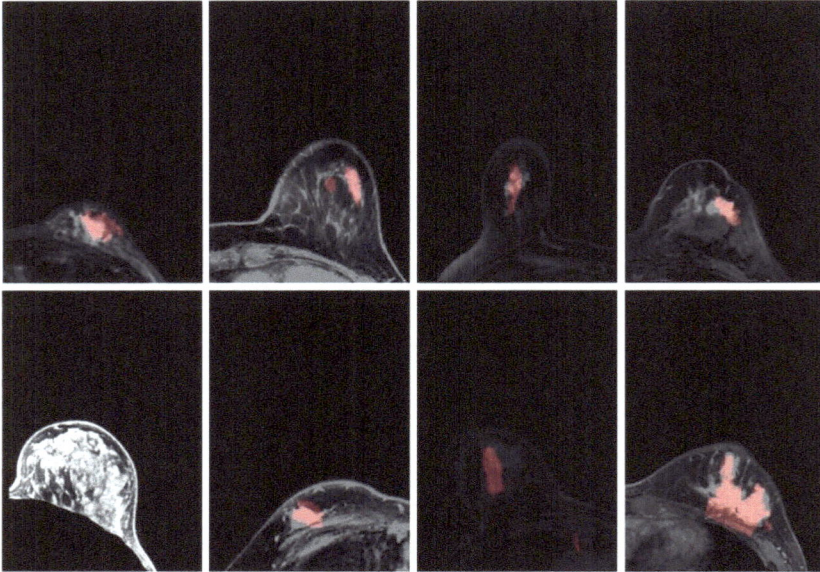

Fig. (4). The registered PET/MR image, with lesions marked as red in the PET image.

4.2. Performance Analysis

A comparison between our method and those of previous studies is shown in Table **3**. The target registration errors of both the fibro-glandular and fat tissues were smaller when determined by our method compared to the results of earlier studies.

Table 3. A comparison of the target registration error (TRE).

	Our Method	**Han *et al.* [2]**	**Hopp *et al.* [18]**
TRE(g)/mm	8.27±2.87	5.12±1.93, 8.36±3.75, 13.53±3.89, 19.54±3.68, 20.38±6.75	11.0±8.3
tre(l)/mm	4.77±2.20		
TRErel	0.19±0.12		0.73±0.90

The high accuracy of registration indicated that our established breast mechanical model has the ability to simulate deformation of the breast from supine to prone. This proposed model fits tissue properties into a complex human tissue model. The application of this model is not restricted to image registration; it can also be used to enhance image guided surgery, breast plastic surgery, and medical device development.

5. CONCLUSION

A patient-specific biomechanical breast model has been established in this project. A stress release method was used to estimate the reference state of the breast, which was straightforward and reliable. Eight pairs of images were used to evaluate the model. The average target error in the eight pairs of images was 8.27±2.87 mm for fibro-glandular tissue and 4.77±2.20 mm for the lesion. The performance of this model was better than that of previous studies. The advantage of this method is that the application is not limited to PET/MR image registration but any deformation from supine to prone. The established patient-specific breast mechanical model can accurately register breasts in the supine position to the prone position. It can also help in the early detection of breast cancer and has the potential to improve radiotherapy planning.

ETHICS APPROVAL

This study was approved by the Human Subjects Ethics Sub-committee of Hong Kong Polytechnic University. The need for written informed consent from the patients was waived, because of the study's retrospective nature. Patient records/information was anonymized and de-identified prior to analysis.

CONFLICT OF INTEREST

The author(s) confirm that this chapter contents have no conflict of interest.

ACKNOWLEDGEMENTS

This work was supported by the Hong Kong Polytechnic University.

REFERENCES

[1]   Cancer Facts & Figures 2016 Atlanta: American Cancer Society. 2016.

[2]   Han L, Hipwell JH, Tanner C, *et al.* Development of patient-specific biomechanical models for predicting large breast deformation. Phys Med Biol 2012; 57(2): 455-72.
[http://dx.doi.org/10.1088/0031-9155/57/2/455] [PMID: 22173131]

[3]   Zienkiewicz OC. The finite element method. 3rd edition. London: McGraw-hill 1977; vol. 3.

[4]   Samani A, Bishop J, Yaffe MJ, Plewes DB. Biomechanical 3-D finite element modeling of the human breast using MRI data. IEEE Trans Med Imaging 2001; 20(4): 271-9.
[http://dx.doi.org/10.1109/42.921476] [PMID: 11370894]

[5]   Gamage TPB, Rajagopal V, Nielsen PM, Nash MP. Patient-specific modeling of breast biomechanics with applications to breast cancer detection and treatment.Patient-Specific Modeling in Tomorrow's Medicine. Springer 2011; pp. 379-412.
[http://dx.doi.org/10.1007/8415_2011_92]

[6]   del Palomar AP, Calvo B, Herrero J, López J, Doblaré M. A finite element model to accurately predict real deformations of the breast. Med Eng Phys 2008; 30(9): 1089-97.
[http://dx.doi.org/10.1016/j.medengphy.2008.01.005] [PMID: 18329940]

[7]   Pathmanathan P, Gavaghan DJ, Whiteley JP, Chapman SJ, Brady JM. Predicting tumor location by modeling the deformation of the breast. IEEE Trans Biomed Eng 2008; 55(10): 2471-80.
[http://dx.doi.org/10.1109/TBME.2008.925714] [PMID: 18838373]

[8]   Azar FS, Metaxas DN, Schnall MD. A finite element model of the breast for predicting mechanical deformations during biopsy procedures IEEE Workshop on Mathematical Methods in Biomedical Image Analysis. 38-45.
[http://dx.doi.org/10.1109/MMBIA.2000.852358]

[9]   Kuhlmann M, Fear EC, Ramirez-Serrano A, Federico S. Mechanical model of the breast for the prediction of deformation during imaging. Med Eng Phys 2013; 35(4): 470-8.
[http://dx.doi.org/10.1016/j.medengphy.2012.06.012] [PMID: 22901855]

[10]   Gamage TPB, Boyes R, Rajagopal V, Nielsen PM, Nash MP. Modelling prone to supine breast deformation under gravity loading using heterogeneous finite element models.Computational Biomechanics for Medicine. Springer 2012; pp. 29-38.
[http://dx.doi.org/10.1007/978-1-4614-3172-5_5]

[11]   Rajagopal V. "Modelling breast tissue mechanics under gravity loading," Doctor of Philosophy in Bioengineering. The University of Auckland 2007.

[12]   Pathmanathan P, Gavaghan D, Whiteley J, Brady M, Nash M, Nielsen P, *et al.* Predicting tumour location by simulating large deformations of the breast using a 3D finite element model and nonlinear elasticity In: Barillot C, Haynor D R, Hellier P, Eds. Medical Image Computing and Computer-Assisted Intervention7th International Conference. Saint-Malo, France. Berlin, Heidelberg: Springer 2004; pp. September 26-29, 2004; 217-24.
[http://dx.doi.org/10.1007/978-3-540-30136-3_28]

[13]   Antoch G, Bockisch A. Combined PET/MRI: a new dimension in whole-body oncology imaging? Eur J Nucl Med Mol Imaging 2009; 36 (Suppl. 1): S113-20.
[http://dx.doi.org/10.1007/s00259-008-0951-6] [PMID: 19104802]

[14]   Unlu MZ, Król A, Magri A, *et al.* Computerized method for nonrigid MR-to-PET breast-image registration. Comput Biol Med 2010; 40(1): 37-53.
[http://dx.doi.org/10.1016/j.compbiomed.2009.10.010] [PMID: 19942214]

[15]   Studholme C, Hill DL, Hawkes DJ. Automated three-dimensional registration of magnetic resonance and positron emission tomography brain images by multiresolution optimization of voxel similarity measures. Med Phys 1997; 24(1): 25-35.
[http://dx.doi.org/10.1118/1.598130] [PMID: 9029539]

[16]   Bezdek JC, Ehrlich R, Full W. FCM: The fuzzy c-means clustering algorithm. Comput Geosci 1984; 10: 191-203.
[http://dx.doi.org/10.1016/0098-3004(84)90020-7]

[17]   Lorensen WE, Cline HE. Marching cubes: A high resolution 3D surface construction algorithmACM siggraph computer graphics. 1987; pp. 163-9.
[http://dx.doi.org/10.1145/37401.37422]

[18]   Hopp T, Dietzel M, Baltzer PA, *et al.* Automatic multimodal 2D/3D breast image registration using biomechanical FEM models and intensity-based optimization. Med Image Anal 2013; 17(2): 209-18.
[http://dx.doi.org/10.1016/j.media.2012.10.003] [PMID: 23265802]

[19]   Azar FS, Metaxas DN, Schnall MD. A deformable finite element model of the breast for predicting mechanical deformations under external perturbations. Acad Radiol 2001; 8(10): 965-75.
[http://dx.doi.org/10.1016/S1076-6332(03)80640-2] [PMID: 11699849]

[20]   Rajagopal V, Chung J, Nielsen P, Nash M. Finite element modelling of breast biomechanics: Finding a reference state IEEE Engineering in Medicine and Biology 27th Annual Conference. 3268-71.
[http://dx.doi.org/10.1109/IEMBS.2005.1617174]

[21]   Bonet J, Wood RD. Nonlinear continuum mechanics for finite element analysis. Cambridge university

press 1997.

[22]   Chung JH, Rajagopal V, Nielsen PM, Nash MP. A biomechanical model of mammographic compressions. Biomech Model Mechanobiol 2008; 7(1): 43-52. [http://dx.doi.org/10.1007/s10237-006-0074-6] [PMID: 17211616]

[23]   Chung J-H. Modelling mammographic mechanics.Doctor of Philosophy. Auckland Bioengineering Institute, The University of Auckland 2008.

[24]   Hibbett, Karlsson, and Sorensen, ABAQUS/standard: User's Manual vol. 1, 1998.

[25]   Rajagopal V, Chung J, Nielsen PM, Nash MP. Finite element modelling of breast biomechanics: directly calculating the reference state. Conf Proc IEEE Eng Med Biol Soc 2006; 1: 420-3. [http://dx.doi.org/10.1109/IEMBS.2006.260047] [PMID: 17946399]

[26]   Lee AW, Schnabel JA, Rajagopal V, Nielsen PM, Nash MP. Breast image registration by combining finite elements and free-form deformations In: Martí J, Oliver A, Freixenet J, Martí R, Eds. 10th International Workshop, IWDM 2010. Girona. June 16-18, 2010; 736-43. [http://dx.doi.org/10.1007/978-3-642-13666-5_99]

Advanced Imaging Analytic Tools for Risk Stratification of Alzheimer's Disease

Abstract: Alzheimer disease (AD) is a neurological disorder characterized by mild cognitive impairment and affects an individual's quality of life. In this chapter, we explore two sets of advanced imaging analytic tools for quantitative detection of the important indicators of AD such as presence of White Matters Hyperintensities and diminished hippocampus. Case studies are used to further illustrate the scope of the use of these tools.

Keywords: Alzheimer Disease, Analytic Tools, Hippocampus, Mild Cognitive Impairment, Risk Stratification, White Matters Hyperintensities.

1. BACKGROUND

Alzheimer's disease (AD), a neurological disorder which is characterized by a decline in cognitive function that affects an individual's daily life. Mild cognitive impairment (MCI) describes the intermediate stage between the expected cognitive decline of normal aging and the more pronounced decline of dementia. Although individual with MCI shows greater problems in memory, language, thinking and judgment than typical age-related retardation, their daily life is usually not affected [1]. Nevertheless, individuals with MCI tend to have an increased risk of developing AD, with the help of new advanced imaging analytic tools, clinicians could diagnose and monitor the progress of people with declining cognitive function [2].

White matter hyperintensities (WMHs) are high intensity signals that appear as white patches in T2 FLAIR images of MRI because WMHs show a larger T2 relaxation rate as a result of an increased tissue water content and degradation of myelin [3]. The presence of WMH is an age-related and genetic problem, which is commonly found in the MR brain among elderly and in people with neurological or vascular disease [4]. WMH will also appear to be more diffusing on MR images of individuals with AD. Nonetheless, individuals with increased expression of apolipoprotein E gene (APOE-Ɛ4) have a higher risk of WMH [5] and facilitate the aggregation of Amyloid-β protein and deposition of plaques in

Fuk-hay Tang

neurons [6]. Also, the thickening and sclerosis of arterial small vessel [7] ischemia and demyelinating disorder [8] will promote the development of WMH.

During healthy aging, there will be unavoidable changes in our brain such as reduction in size and increase in WHH patches though they appear in much later age for some people. However, the cortical part of the brain that responsible for thinking, planning and remembering shrivels up a lot more on the individual with AD. Shrinkage is especially severe in the hippocampus, which plays a main role in forming new memories. Oppositely, fluid-filled spaces within the brain known as ventricles will grow a lot larger too [2]. Therefore, the quantitative assessment of hippocampus, ventricles and WMH volumes acts as important predictors of early AD. In this regard, we aim to illustrate the use of two sets of advanced imaging analytic tools for the segmentation and quantitative detection of the presence of WMH and diminished hippocampus volume through case studies.

2. SEGMENTATION AND QUANTITATIVE DETECTION OF WMH

WMH is usually found in the perivascular spaces and periventricular white matter [9] (Haller, Kövari& Herrmann, 2013), and mainly involve the frontal lobe (70%) and parietal lobe (22%) [10] thus affects one's cognitive function [11]. However, although it has high sensitivity, its specificity is limited by the numerous possible indication of WMH such as existence of lacunar infarcts, micro-hemorrhages and small vessel cerebrovascular disease [5].

In order to detect the presence and volumetric changes in WMH during the transformation under different cognitive statuses, MATLAB, SPM12, W2MHS and VBM8 were used to process the collected MR images from the database of previous AD studies including MIDAS, MRBrainS and NACC database. MATLAB, also known as MATrix LABoratory, was used for signal processing and image processing optimization [12]. SPM12 was used for analyzing brain imaging data sequences ranging from fMRI, PET, SPECT, EEG and MEG [13]. MRIcron, a tool for cross-platform NIfTI format image viewer, was for loading multiple layers of images, generating volume rendering and drawing volume of interest [14], while W2MHS, another toolbox known as Wisconsin White Matter Hyperintensities Segmentation Toolbox, was applied for precise segmentation of WMHs and quantification of their effective volume (EV) based on the WMH probability map generated by W2MHS [15]. Last of all, the grey matter (GM), white matter (WM) and cerebro-spinal fluid (CSF) volume were determined by VBM8 toolbox.

In total, 352 cases were analyzed using the method mentioned above. All collected data were then defined into normal or AD group according to the diagnoses provided from the respective database. 93 subjects, ranging from 66 to

95 years old were defined as normal while 259 subjects fell into the AD group. The information about the volume of WMH, GM and WMH of all subjects was collected, and analyzed together with their clinical background (number of APOE alleles and AD progression).

With the help of advanced imaging tool, the effective volume of WMH, GM and WM was found to be increased with age Fig. (**1a** to **1c**). However, the effective volume collected in the present study were lower than that in previous studies, probably due to differences in age and racial groups [16, 17]. As shown in Table **1**, WMH volume was also found to be increased (up to 32% increased) in subjects with MCI and AD after the first year of diagnosis. The clustering of APOE alleles in normal and AD subjects tends to have a higher volume of WMH (Table **2**). In this connection, MCI subjects having at least one APOE allele are highly prone to become AD when compared with the APOE allele (Table **3**). In addition, subjects with two APOE alleles are the most vulnerable to develop AD at around 75 years old.

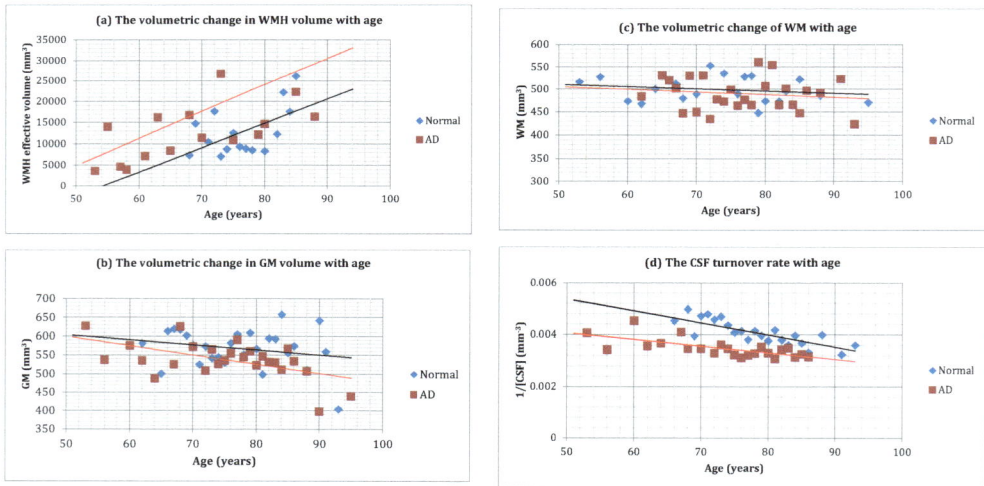

Fig. (1). Volumetric changes in WMH, GM and WM, and CSF turnover rate with age.
(**a**) The volume of WMH in AD was slightly higher than normal individuals at all ages.
From (**b**) to (**d**) show a trend in decreasing volume in Grey matter (GM), volume in white matter (WM) and CSF turnover rate with increasing age.

As indicated in Fig. (**1a**), the volume of GM was found decreased with age at a higher rate in AD subjects. The faster decreasing rate explains why AD subjects have difficulties in carrying out multi-step tasks, learning new things, problems in recognizing etc. providing that grey matter is the component in our brain that is responsible for executing cognitive function and memory. The decreasing rate is slightly similar in the volume of WM but with AD having a lower starting point.

Table 1. The progression of Cognitive status in relation to % change of WMH volume.

	Subjects Diagnosed as MCI		Subjects Diagnosed as AD
	Remains as MCI After 1 Year	**Progressed to AD After a Mean Age of 2.6 Years**	**Remains as AD After a Mean Age of 2.6 Years**
No. of Subjects	2	10	15
% Change of WMH Volume	19.66	18.24	32.12

Table 2. The clustering of APOE alleles in relation to WMH, GM, WM and CSF volumes.

Cognitive Status	No. of APOE Alleles	No. of Subjects	Average Age (Years)	Average WMH (mm³)	Average GM (mm³)	Average WM (mm³)	Average CSF (mm³)
Normal	0	70	88	75	23,934	567.45	493.54	246.46
	1	17			12,773			
	2	1			74,471			
AD	1	111	143	77	2,894	530.344	481.20	286.03
	2	32			16,640			

Table 3. The clustering of APOE alleles in relation to the age of first diagnosis of AD.

Cognitive Status Transformation	No. of APOE Alleles	Age at First AD Diagnosis (Years)	Year Span Between First Medical Consultation and AD Diagnosis	No. of Subjects
MCI→AD	0	82	2.7	49
	1	77	2.0	66
	2	75	3.0	14
N→AD	0	86	6.5	2
	1	79	7.0	1

Furthermore, the turnover rate of CSF also decreased with aging. The main function of the CSF is to transport nutrients and remove wastes to and from the brain. Since the turnover rate in AD subjects is lower than that of normal, the reveal AD subjects have a greater reduction in resistance to oxidative stress, clearing proteins, peptides and other potentially toxic metabolites [18], resulting in increasing chance of brain damage in AD subjects.

3. BRAIN VOLUME ANALYTIC TOOL

NeuroQuant is one of the many commercial imaging tools that can determine brain volume within a reasonable time. The precise measurement of brain volume could help to improve the early detection and treatment of neurodegenerative disorders and AD as they suffer from brain atrophy (shrinkage). This tool automatically segments and measures the volumes of the hippocampus, ventricles and other brain structures and makes comparison among data and norms [19]. Thus, it is a convenient and cost-effective way to get reliable and objective results. Yet, the quantification of the volume of the brain in AD does not pinpoint the exact disease in which the patient is suffering from and quantify WMH volume.

Sixteen subjects ranging from 56 to 92 years old with T1 non-contrast sagittal images from the ADNI database were used for illustration. Their cognitive status was divided into 3 groups, namely Normal, MCI, and AD. From the reports, NeuroQuant failed to quantify WMH volume and inform us nothing about the specific the patient suffered from. Only information about a decrease in the volume of hippocampus and an increase in the ventricles with age were collected among all different cognitive statuses of 16 subjects. Therefore, this imaging tool is more like a general overview of the brain volume instead. In addition, it can help us to compare that subject's volume with the normal reference values Fig. (**2**).

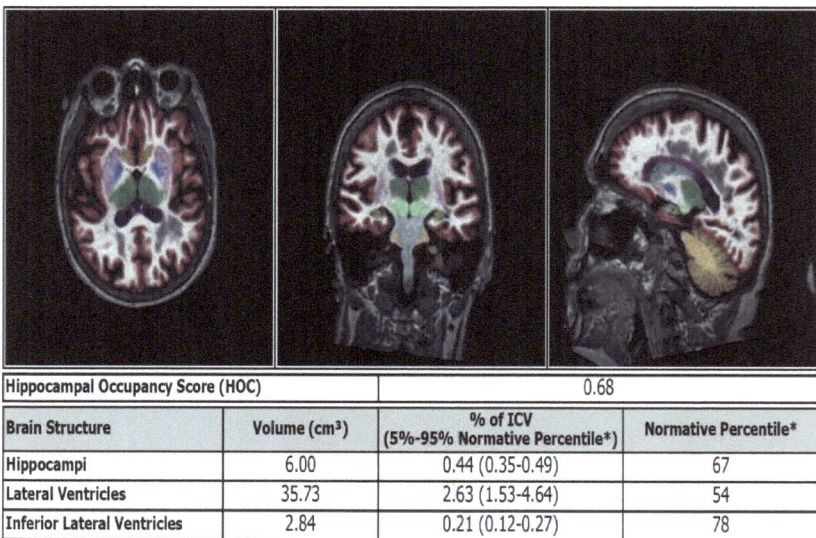

Hippocampal Occupancy Score (HOC)		0.68	
Brain Structure	**Volume (cm³)**	**% of ICV** (5%-95% Normative Percentile*)	**Normative Percentile***
Hippocampi	6.00	0.44 (0.35-0.49)	67
Lateral Ventricles	35.73	2.63 (1.53-4.64)	54
Inferior Lateral Ventricles	2.84	0.21 (0.12-0.27)	78

Fig. (2). NeuroQuant can determine the volume of hippocampi with age-matched reference value for the prediction of AD. Courtesy: screen capture from the NeuroQuant report.

Take one of the generated reports as an example Fig. (**3**). From this report, we can see that the subject's hippocampus volume trend is going from lower 50% to upper 50% (black dot: 72 years old, grey dot: 66 years old). So, approximate estimation of his memory function which is declining in a faster rate than normal can be estimated, implicating that there is an increasing chance of dementia development such as AD and MCI. In fact, the detail report generated by NeuroQuant has reached the quality so as to satisfy both medical professionals and patients. A combination of reports ranging from age related atrophy to triage brain atrophy could be neatly presented in an easily understood format, providing an early and more precise warning to those who started showing early AD signs and symptoms.

AGE-MATCHED REFERENCE CHARTS*

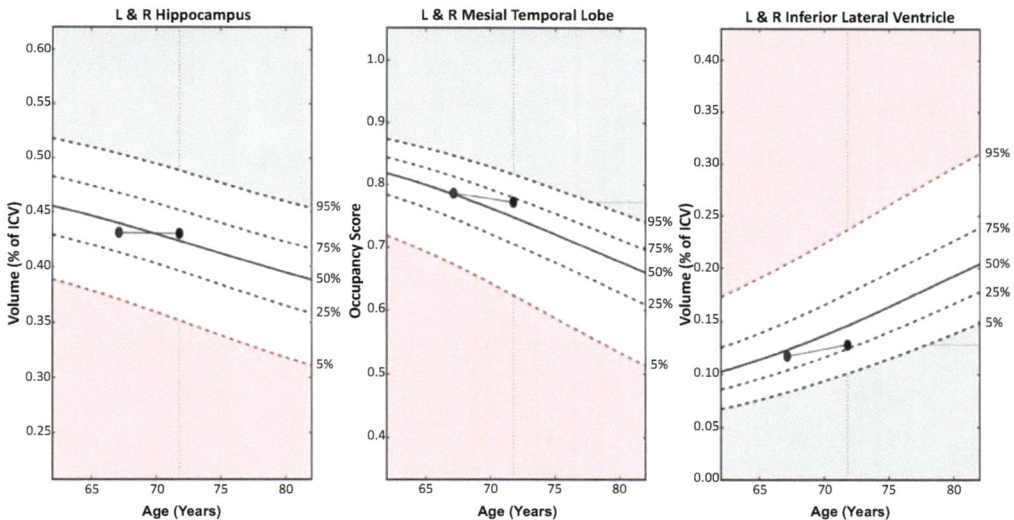

*Charts and normative values are provided for reference purposes only.

Fig. (3). NeuroQuant summaries the volume of hippocampus, mesial temporal lobe and inferior lateral ventricle of a volunteer at the age of 66 (grey dot) and 72 (Black dot), respectively. Courtesy: screen capture from the NeuroQuant report.

4. LIMITATION OF THE PRESENT STUDY

As sample subjects collected from the various AD database for illustration were used, the observed results may not be valid in all situations as more than 90% of our subjects are American. Moreover, sample size may be too small. Further, study using these advanced imaging tools is warranted.

Besides, diminished brain volume and WMH have no definite relationship with suffering from AD. Other differential clinical markers such as the presence of the accumulation of amyloid-β peptide plaques and neurofibrillary tangles should be considered.

5. CONCLUSION

Recently, there is an increasing trend of medical application of advanced imaging tools, worldwide. Besides diagnosing AD, they can also contribute in diagnosing multiple sclerosis, epilepsy and traumatic brain injury. WMH is an increase in MR signal intensity in the brain, and is associated with aging. They can be segmented and quantitatively determined by many imaging tools like W2MHS. There seems to be an increase in WMH volume with the progression of AD when compared to normal subjects. Further correlation analysis reviewed that the clustering of APOE alleles would lead to progression to AD at an earlier age. We also found that there was a greater decrease in GM and WM volume in AD than in normal group. To conclude, we discussed the use of new advanced imaging analytic tools for risk stratification of Alzheimer's disease with illustrative cases in this chapter.

CONFLICT OF INTEREST

The author(s) confirm that this chapter contents have no conflict of interest.

ACKNOWLEDGEMENTS

Declared none

REFERENCES

[1]   2015. What is AD/MCI?. Retrieved August 11, 2016 from http://www.adrc.wisc.edu/what-admci

[2]   2015.Alzheimer's   Changes   the   Brain   Retrieved   August   11,   2015   from https://www.alz.org/braintour/alzheimers_changes.asp

[3]   Jack CR Jr, O'Brien PC, Rettman DW, *et al.* FLAIR histogram segmentation for measurement of leukoaraiosis volume. J Magn Reson Imaging 2001; 14(6): 668-76.
[http://dx.doi.org/10.1002/jmri.10011] [PMID: 11747022]

[4]   DeCarli C, Murphy DG, Tranh M, *et al.* The effect of white matter hyperintensity volume on brain structure, cognitive performance, and cerebral metabolism of glucose in 51 healthy adults. Neurology 1995; 45(11): 2077-84.
[http://dx.doi.org/10.1212/WNL.45.11.2077] [PMID: 7501162]

[5]   Brickman A M, Zahodne L B, Guzman V A. Reconsidering harbingers of dementia: progression of parietal lobe white matter hyperintensities predicts Alzheimer's disease incidence. Neurobiology of Aging, 2014; 36(1): 27-32.

[6]   Holtzman DM, Bales KR, Tenkova T. Apolipoprotein E isoform-dependent amyloid deposition and neuritic degeneration in a mouse model of Alzheimer's disease. *PNAS, 97* (6), 2892–2897. BMJ 2000; 341.

[7]   Huang YH, Zhang WW, Lin L, *et al.* Could changes in arterioles impede the perivascular drainage of

interstitial fluid from the cerebral white matter in leukoaraiosis? Neuropathol Appl Neurobiol 2010; 36(3): 237-47.
[http://dx.doi.org/10.1111/j.1365-2990.2009.01049.x] [PMID: 19889176]

[8]   Pantoni L, Garcia JH. Pathogenesis of leukoaraiosis: a review. Stroke 1997; 28(3): 652-9.
[http://dx.doi.org/10.1161/01.STR.28.3.652] [PMID: 9056627]

[9]   Haller S, Kövari E, Herrmann FR, *et al.* Do brain T2/FLAIR white matter hyperintensities correspond to myelin loss in normal aging? A radiologic-neuropathologic correlation study. Acta Neuropathol Commun 2013; 1(14): 14.
[http://dx.doi.org/10.1186/2051-5960-1-14] [PMID: 24252608]

[10]   Capizzano AA, Ación L, Bekinschtein T, *et al.* White matter hyperintensities are significantly associated with cortical atrophy in Alzheimer's disease. J Neurol Neurosurg Psychiatry 2004; 75(6): 822-7.
[http://dx.doi.org/10.1136/jnnp.2003.019273] [PMID: 15145992]

[11]   Gunning-Dixon FM, Raz N. The cognitive correlates of white matter abnormalities in normal aging: a quantitative review. Neuropsychology 2000; 14(2): 224-32.
[http://dx.doi.org/10.1037/0894-4105.14.2.224] [PMID: 10791862]

[12]   Sandberg K, Wright G. Introduction to MATLAB Retrieved July 10 2013.

[13]   Guillaume S. 2014. SPM. Retrieved July 10, 2016 from http://www.fil.ion.ucl.ac.uk/spm/

[14]   Vendemia S, Hanayik T, Rorden C. 2014. NITRC: MRIcron. Retrieved July 10, 2016 from https://www.nitrc.org/projects/mricron

[15]   Lindner C, Ithapu V. 2014. NITRC: Wisconsin White Matter Hyperintensities Segmentation Toolbox. Retrieved July 10, 2016 from https://www.nitrc.org/projects/w2mhs/

[16]   Atwood LD, Wolf PA, Heard-costa NL. Genetic Variation in White Matter Hyperintensity Volume in the Framingham Study 2004; 35: 1609-13.

[17]   Luders E, Steinmetz H, Jancke L. Brain size and grey matter volume in the healthy human brain. Cognitive Neuroscience and Neuropsychology 2002; 13(17)

[18]   Chiu C, Miller M C, Caralopoulos L N. Science. Temporal course of cerebrospinal fluid dynamics and amyloid accumulation in the aging rat brain from three to thirty months 2012; 9(3)

[19]   2015.CorTechs Labs NeuroQuant Retrieved July 13, 2016 from http://www.cortechslabs.com/neuroquant/

Recent Advances in Imaging, 2018, *Vol. 1*, 53-82

CHAPTER 7

Imaging Beyond Bone Mineral Density

Abstract: Bone is a composite tissue comprised of organic and inorganic phases. It adapts itself to mechanical strains with an aim to maintain its mechanical competence *via* modelling and remodeling. Such adaptation of bone can result in alteration of material and structural properties including bone mineral density (BMD), micro-architecture, mineralization, and morphology. Quantitative bone imaging enables the evaluation of bone status in relation to diseases, mechanical and other interventions. However, bone quantity measurement of BMD using dual-energy X-Ray absorptiometry is limited because of its projection imaging approach and provides only a scalar measurement. As an anisotropic material, other bone quality including the architecture and spatial distribution of bone have to be considered in the evaluation of bone status. Also collagen fiber orientation and degree of mineralization in this composite tissue are important determinants of bone adaptation in response to treatment interventions. Thus, synergized use of multi-imaging modalities may decipher the interplay of material and structural properties in bone adaptation. Current imaging techniques using peripheral quantitative computed tomography, micro-computed tomography, magnetic resonance imaging, quantitative ultrasound and circularly polarized light microscopic imaging have gone beyond the measurement of bone quantity and to provide significant information of bone quality in the understanding of bone status. The present chapter aims to discuss the contribution of different imaging modalities in the evaluation of bone status.

Keywords: Bone Quantity, Bone Quality, Bone Strength, Imaging.

1. IMAGING BEYOND BONE MINERAL DENSITY

The bone strength is determined by both the material and structural properties, which are regulated by the activities of bone modelling and bone remodelling (Fig. **1**). The former is responsible for the bone growth while the latter is for the maintenance of bone balance [1]. In accordance with the Utah paradigm of bone physiology, mechanical loading is the main driving force, *via* bone modelling and remodelling in the maintenance of bone competence to the demand of loading and metabolism, with the mediation of other non-mechanical factors, such as, nutrition, hormones and cytokines [2]. Imaging has provided a valuable asset in the non-invasive/non-destructive assessment of bone mineral density (BMD), bone macrostructure and microstructure [3 - 8], degree of mineralization [9 - 11], collagen fibre [12] and microdamage [13, 14].

Fuk-hay Tang

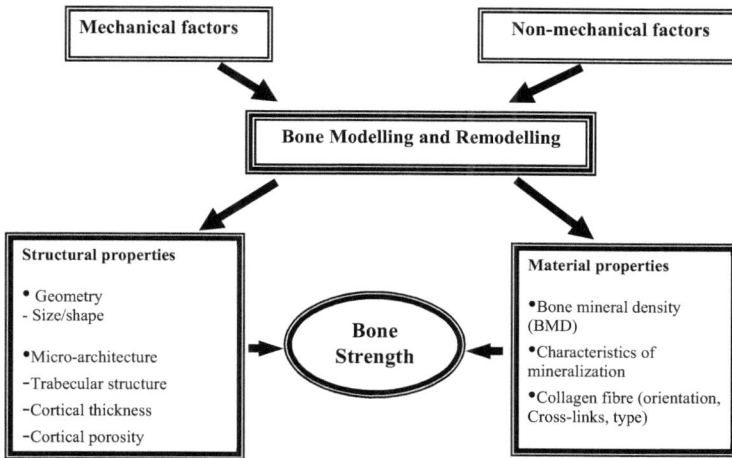

Fig. (1). Dependence of bone mechanical strength in relation to its structural and material properties, mediated by bone modelling and remodelling in response to mechanical and non-mechanical factors (adapted from [15]).

1.1. Imaging of Trabecular Bone Micro-Architecture

Numerous studies have demonstrated that trabecular bone micro-architecture accounts for a significant variance in the explanation of bone strength [15 - 20] and performs better when combined with BMD in the discrimination of patients with and without osteoporotic fractures [21 - 24]. Currently, there are several imaging techniques including conventional radiography, quantitative ultrasound, quantitative magnetic resonance imaging and computed tomography allow quantification of trabecular bone structure.

1.1.1. Conventional Radiography

Semi-quantitative analysis of trabecular pattern in proximal femur radiograph using Singh index was employed to quantify the degree of bone loss [25]. However, the method is subject to intra and inter-observer variability. Quantification of the complexity and spatial distribution of the trabecular bone texture can be achieved using fractal analyses. The use of conventional radiographs for such analyses requires film quality control including standardization of the film-screen combination, selection of exposure parameters and use of calibration phantom that fractal dimensions as estimated in the radiographs can be reliably compared [26, 27]. In an *in vitro* study, conventional radiography and fractal analysis were used to quantify trabecular texture patterns in radiographs of human femur specimens in conjunction with BMD measured by quantitative computed tomography (QCT) to predict bone strength. Using multivariate regression analysis, fractal dimension combined with BMD improved the correlations with biomechanical properties (r= 0.77 to 0.83) [28]. In an *in vivo* study employing fractal analysis on calcaneus radiographs, the fractal dimension allows a significant diagnostic performance (area under the receiver operating curve (AUC) = 0.824) in the differentiation of osteoporotic patients with vertebral crush fracture compared to femoral neck BMD (AUC = 0.633).

1.1.2. Quantitative Ultrasound

Since the pioneering work by Langton and Palmer *et al.*, quantitative ultrasound (QUS) has been developed for the assessment of skeletal status [29]. Current ultrasound scanners are applicable to calcaneum (Fig. **2**), patella, radius and tibia.

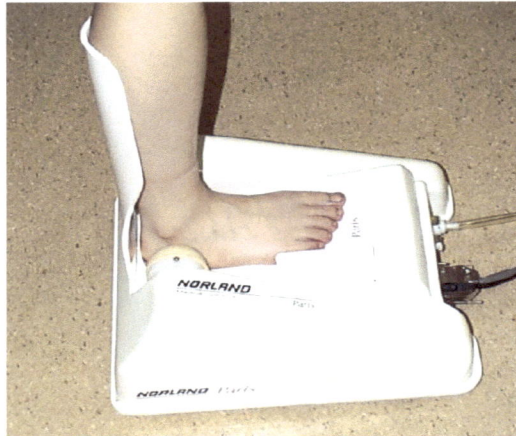

Fig. (2). Calcaneal bone ultrasonometer (Courtesy: Bone Quality and Health Centre, Department of Orthopaedics and Traumatology, The Chinese University of Hong Kong).

Ultrasound has the advantages such as being non-ionizing, the system is portable and relatively inexpensive. As such, QUS may be more useful than BMD in population-based study. The calcaneum is the most common measurement site due to its accessibility, suitable shape, and high trabecular content [30, 31]. Early experience suggests that ultrasound measurement parameters, namely broadband ultrasound attenuation (BUA) and speed of sound (SOS) provide information not only about bone density but also about architecture and elasticity [32, 33]. Calcaneal trabecular BMD alone explained 88-93% of variance in SOS whereas BMD combined with elasticity and anisotropic variables explained 96-98% of the variance in SOS [34]. In another study by Hodgskinson and Njeh *et al.* showed similar results with improved prediction when combining ultrasound velocity and apparent density [35]. Precision of BUA measurements (% coefficient of variation

(CV)) ranges from 2% to 5% while that of velocity is typically 0.5% to 1.5% [36]. Calcaneal ultrasound densitometer with imaging devices allows standardization of measurement of region of interest in patients which may improve precision.

Correlation study in 109 elderly aged 65-87 showed that Calcaneal BUA showed higher correlations with BMD (measured by dual-energy X-ray absorptiometry (DXA)) values of the lumbar spine, femoral neck, trochanter and total body than calcaneal and tibial SOS (r = 0.48-0.64, r = 0.30-0.47, r = 0.35-0.47, respectively, $P < 0.001$) [37]. Another study in 209 postmenopausal women demonstrated that when SOS, BUA and Stiffness were regressed against lumbar spine BMD and femoral BMD as measured by DXA and the correlation coefficients were in the range 0.52-0.58 [38]. A recent study showed that BUA, velocity of sound (VOS) and Soundness measured by calcaneal QUS were significantly correlated with trabecular BMD, cortical BMD and integrated BMD of both distal tibia and distal radius measured by pQCT (r = 0.210-0.447, $P < 0.01$) [39]. These studies illustrate that there is modest correlation between these QUS parameters and BMD measurement because they may measure different properties of the bone. It follows that the use of QUS as a surrogate for BMD measurement may not be feasible. However, several prospective studies have shown that ultrasound measurement employing water-based foot placement in calcaneum is as effective as DXA in predicting risk of hip fracture [40, 41], and the predictability is independent of the bone mineral density. It is likely that both modalities are complementary to each other in the prediction of fracture risk. Cross-sectional study in Korean by Kim and Kim *et al.* shows that the risk factors associated with low quantitative ultrasound values are similar to that of low bone mass [42]. Thus, QUS can be used as pre-screening tool [43, 44] to identify high risk patients and then be referred for further examination by bone densitometric methods. Clinical risk factors can provide with an indication of bone mass status whereas QUS parameters, in addition to that, reflect the bone structure and elasticity. Composite strategy employing a model constituting clinical risk factors and QUS parameters may become advantageous. As such, it may allow primary care physicians with limited access to bone densitometry, the possibility to select high-risk patients for follow up. In a population-based study of 2387 women, it showed that QUS worked as well as central DXA in identifying women at high risk of prevalent vertebral fracture [45].

Previous numerous exercise intervention studies using the preferred technique DXA have demonstrated an osteogenic effect [46 - 50]. However, DXA scan in these studies only measures bone status in terms of BMD, not bone structure. Techniques such as bone histomorphometry and microCT are used for direct quantitative study of bone micro-architecture but they are invasive. Use of QUS can serve as an alternative to reveal indirectly the osteogenic response in terms of alteration of bone micro-architecture. The application of such has been illustrated in a cross-sectional study on male sportsman aged 18-22 by Yung and Lai *et al.* which demonstrated that swimming exercise, a non-weight bearing activity brought about higher calcaneal BUA (3.5-5.6%) and velocity of sound (VOS) (3.0-3.4%) compared with the sedentary control [51]. This concurs with the study in prepubertal and early-pubertal female athletes by Falk and Bronshtein *et al.* that swimming exercise enhanced bone properties with high tibial SOS [52]. Thus swimming, a non-weight bearing exercise, which is believed to have an insignificant effect on bone density, may have favorable effects on bone properties such as elasticity and microstructure, which are detectable in QUS but not in DXA.

1.1.3. Quantitative Magnetic Resonance Imaging

Hydrogen protons are abundant in human tissues. Applying an external magnetic field generated by a magnetic resonance imaging (MRI) scanner, the hydrogen protons align with the magnetic field and the magnetic axis of proton sweeps out a cone. This movement is called precession. To produce an MR image, the hydrogen protons are excited with a radiofrequency (RF) pulse. Exposure of these protons to radiofrequency (RF) pulse causes their magnetic axis to swing through either 90° or 180° depending on the pulse sequence. When the RF pulse is off, the protons will again turn to process in alignment with the external magnetic field. This is known as relaxation and in doing so, it produces an RF signal which can be detected on RF coils. By using the signal information, the density of proton and the time it takes to turn can be used for quantitative analyses and to establish an MR image [53].

In quantitative MR, the apparent bone marrow transverse relaxation time T2* is measured, the differences in magnetic tissue parameters between the trabecular bone structure and bone marrow content produce a distortion of the local magnetic field that influences the relaxation time, which depends on the density of the trabecular network and its geometry [4, 7]. A well connected and complex trabecular bone exhibits shorter T2* compared with loosely connected trabecular bone. *In vivo* precision of T2* in repeated bone marrow measurements at distal radius and calcaneus ranges from 3.8%-9.5% CV [54] and 4%-10% CV [7], respectively.

Experimental studies demonstrated a reduction in T2* of both water and cottonseed oil in the presence of bone power using MR spectroscopy [55] and water present in the trabecular spaces compared to extratrabecular water using high field spectroscopy at 5.88 Tesla [56]. These properties allow quantitative MR applied in studying trabecular bone architecture and assessing osteoporosis.

Spatial change in relaxation rate, $1/T2^*$ was shown as a function of distance from the joint endplate. This corresponds to greatest bone density at the epiphyses and decreases towards the metaphysis and diaphysis [57]. This concurs with the study by Lai and Qin *et al*. that the regional trabecular BMD as measured by pQCT in both ultradistal radius and ultradistal tibia showed a significant linear trend decline from the distal to proximal aspects ($P < 0.001$) [58]. As suggested by the latter study, this increased tBMD combined with increased bone area towards the bone joint endplate may adapt to withstand the axial impact loading.

MR imaging of trabecular bone structure is non-invasive and allows direct multi-planar image acquisition (Fig. **3**). Applications of quantitative MR imaging in bone morphology have been found in peripheral anatomical sites, such as distal radius, calcaneum and phalanges in view of the constraints of spatial resolution and acquisition time to obtain sufficient image signal-to-noise ratio. The acquired MR image is first binarized separating the trabecular bone from the bone marrow. The segmentation has defied challenges in MR image as compared to CT image because relatively more technical factors affecting the MR image quality have to be optimized. This can include field strength, pulse sequence (spin echo verse gradient echo sequences), echo time, repetition time, RF coils and thresholding algorithms [59]. From this binarized image, the morphologic parameters such as apparent bone volume fraction (App.BV/TV), apparent trabecular thickness (App.Tb.Th), apparent trabecular separation (App.Tb.Sp) and apparent trabecular number (App.Tb.N), similar to those of the standard histomorphometry are then derived with model based (plate model) mean intercept length methods or model independent, distance transformation algorithms [60]. Fractal analysis can also be applied to the binarized image to obtain fractal dimension which demonstrates the ability to discriminate osteoporotic hip fractures and control in earlier studies [61]. Morphometric parameters derived from the MR image at a slice thickness that is comparable with the dimension of a trabecular bone (100-150 μm) are subject to partial volume effect. Thus true estimation of BV/TV, Tb.Th. Tb.N and Tb.Sp using MR image at 1.5 Telsa and 3.0 Telsa was not demonstrated when compared to that of micro-computed tomography (microCT) [60] and contact radiography macro-section [23] as the reference. Nevertheless, there were significant correlations of morphologic parameters derived from these imaging modalities. Recent study in the use of microMRI in mice with gradient echo pulse sequence acquired both ex vivo and *in vivo* (resolution: 35 x 35 x 200 μm, 11.7 Telsa field strength) was demonstrated to be comparable to histology in terms of cortical bone thickness, percentage area of trabecular bone and marrow [62].

Morphologic parameters derived from high resolution MR images of cadaveric bone samples combined with BMD measurements have been shown to improve the prediction of mechanical competence [63 - 67]. For example, cadaveric femoral bone cubes, n=32 (resolution: 117 x 156 x 300 μm, 1.5 Tesla field strength) combined with QCT measured BMD improved the prediction of maximum compressive strength with a significant increase in variance from 0.79 to 0.88 [63]. Morphological and textural parameters derived from *in vivo* MR images of calcaneus and radius have shown the ability to discriminate patients with and without spine and hip fractures [24, 61, 68 - 70]. For examples the study by Link and Majumdar *et al.* showed that using calcaneal MR image to derive morphological measures, App.Tb.Sp, App.Tb.N and App. BV/TV achieve the strongest discriminators and the highest diagnostic performance in differentiating patients with and without osteoporotic hip fractures, with the values of AUC at 0.78, 0.77 and 0.73, respectively [61]. In another study by Wehrli and Gomberg *et al.* employed a novel approach, digital topological analysis (DTA), to create a skeletonization of the radius MR image. The skeletonized images contain only surfaces, profiles, curves, and their mutual junctions as the remnants of trabecular plates and rods after skeletonization [69]. DTA parameters were the strongest discriminators between subjects with and without spinal deformities compared with integral BMD in the lumbar spine and femur as well as MR-derived BV/TV. Subjects with deformities (n = 29) had lower topological surface (SURF) density (p < 0.0005) and surface-to-curve ratio (SCR; a measure of the ratio of plate like to rod like trabeculae; p < 0.0005) than those without. Profile interior (PI) density, a measure of intact trabecular rods, was also lower in the deformity group (p < 0.0001) [69].

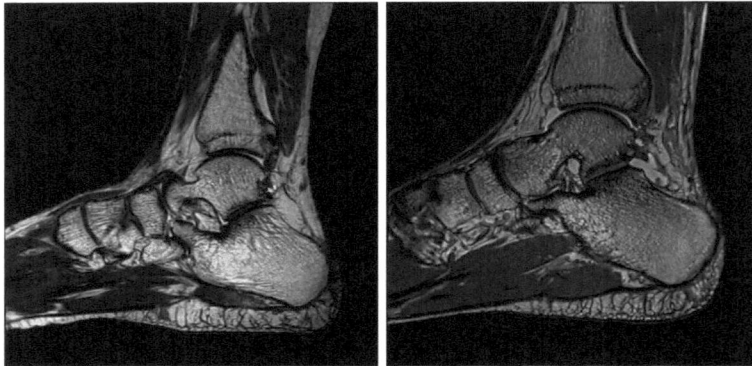

Fig. (3). 1.5 T(left) and 3.0 T (right) MRI sagittal view of heel bone showing better detail of rabecular pattern in 3.0 T scan.

Other applications of MR imaging in studying bone quality at biochemical level including spectroscopy, and perfusion imaging which enable quantitative evaluation of marrow fat content and blood perfusion in bone marrow, respectively. Fat content quantification in phantom study using different MR imaging techniques, with reference to MR spectroscopy, including chemical shift saturation (r^2 = 0.938), opposed-phase saturation (r^2= 0.88) and iterative decomposition of water and fat with echo asymmetry and least-square estimation (IDEAL) (r^2= 0.985) demonstrated a high accuracy of these imaging techniques [71]. Bone with increased fat fraction may compromise with its resistance to fracture as it is more compressible than haematopoietic tissue [72]. Studies showed that average fat content was significantly elevated in patients with osteoporosis/osteopenia compared with controls [73 - 75]. Griffith, Yeung *et al.* demonstrated a link between bone blood flow, marrow fat and osteoporosis using proton MR spectroscopy and dynamic contrast-enhanced MR imaging. Significant decreased in marrow perfusion with increased marrow fat content in proximal femur and lumbar spine were demonstrated in subjects with osteoporosis compared to subjects with osteopenia [76 - 78].

1.1.4. Computed Tomography

Computed tomography (CT) employs a narrow X-ray beam scanning around the object. Differential attenuation of X-ray beam occurs depending on the object absorption coefficients which are a function of its physical density, thickness and atomic number. The transmitted X-ray beam carrying the signal information is received by the data acquisition system. The latter converts the X-ray signals into digital formation. By which the computer reconstructs the image using back projection method. This results in a cross-sectional image that composes of an array of pixels. The digital image data lends itself well to computer manipulation so that multi-planar reformation and three-dimensional (3D) voxel image reconstruction can be achieved [79]. Currently, several approaches can be used to quantify bone morphology. This includes quantitative computed tomography (QCT), peripheral computed tomography (pQCT), microCT and synchrotron CT [80].

Both QCT and pQCT allows determination of axial and appendicular skeletal true volumetric bone mineral density, respectively, and separate evaluation of cortical and trabecular bone (Fig. **4**). The latter is advantageous in that differential response of trabecular as opposed to cortical bone to treatment intervention, senile and oestrogen-related bone loss can be monitored [81 - 85]. QCT employs clinical CT scanner with improved in-plane resolution of 0.2 mm when using multi-slice spiral CT compared to 0.5 mm achieved with conventional CT scanner [4, 19, 23]. Nevertheless, the minimal slice thickness ranging from 0.5-1.0 mm predisposes the image to partial volume effect. Added to that, the polychromatic X-ray beam contributes to beam hardening effect. The latter creates streak artefacts and together with the partial volume effect attribute to misrepresentation of the image [86]. Thus, similar to high resolution MR image, the high resolution CT image derived morphologic parameters are subject to bias. Recent studies by Link and

Vieth *et al.* showed that high resolution (0.152 x 0.153 x 0.9 mm) MR-derived structure parameters performed better in the prediction of trabecular bone structure compared to that of multi-slice spiral CT (0.247 x 0.247 x 1 mm) [23]. Nevertheless, CT imaging at the peripheral site has added advantages. The peripheral location of the human tibia and radius, with its relatively small amount of surrounding tissue increases the accuracy and the precision of BMD measurements due to a reduction in the beam hardening effect and negligible soft tissue correction [87]. Multi-slice pQCT measures the tBMD, the integral BMD (iBMD) at the ultradistal radius/tibia, and the cortical BMD (cBMD) at its distal site [82, 88]. Such studies have reported that pQCT is highly reproducible, with a coefficient of variation (CV) of 0.25-0.4% for such *in vivo* BMD measurements. As such, a low-precision error allows an accurate baseline and follow-up study of inter- and intra-skeletal site comparisons of volumetric BMD [58, 84, 89, 90]. Volumetric trabecular BMD of human vertebral specimens as measured by pQCT (in plane resolution: 0.11 mm) in combination with apparent trabecular connectivity measures derived by skeletonization of the images improved the prediction of elastic modulus ($r^2 = 0.86$, $p < 0.01$) [91]. A later study with similar pQCT image resolution by Wachter and August demonstrated no significant improvement in the prediction of elastic modulus, strength and maximum energy absorption when combining vBMD and apparent trabecular morphological parameters measured at the intertrochanteric region of proximal femur [92]. This could be attributed to the skeletal site difference in which the trabecular structure of proximal femur is more heterogeneous and that decreases the predictive value of structural parameters [92]. The pQCT scanner (Densiscan 2000, Scanco Medical, Bassersdorf, Switzerland) used in the studies by Lai and Qin *et al* has got 300 μm in plane resolution and 1 mm slice thickness, the depiction of trabecular bone architecture is not adequate [58, 93, 94]. Recent advance in high resolution pQCT (HR-pQCT) scanner design (10% MTF, isotropic voxel size 82 μm) (Fig. **5a**, **b**) allows high resolution *in vivo* imaging study of micro-architectural features in radius and tibia in addition to volumetric BMD [95].

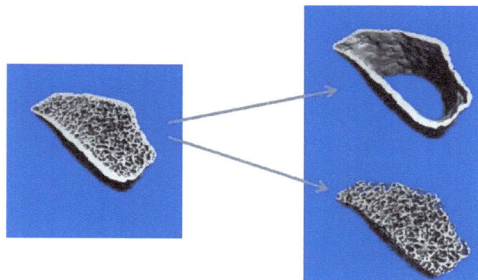

Fig. (4). Segmentation of cortical and trabecular bone for separate evaluation. (Courtesy: Bone Quality and Health Centre, Department of Orthopaedics and Traumatology, The Chinese University of Hong Kong).

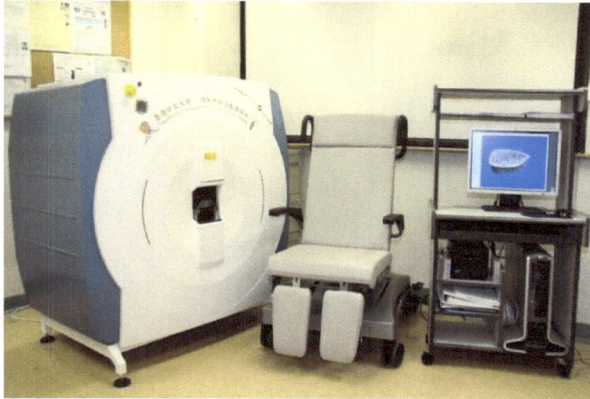

Fig. (5a). *In vivo* High resolution pQCT for extremities.

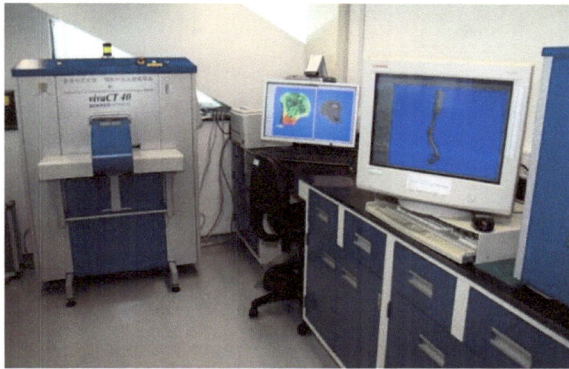

Fig. (5b). High resolution pQCT showing normal verse osteoporotic bone in distal tibia (Courtesy: Bone Quality and Health Centre, Department of Orthopaedics and Traumatology, The Chinese University of Hong Kong).

The microCT system was first introduced by Feldkamp *et al.* who employed a microfocus cone beam X-ray tube and a two dimensional image intensifier as a detector to produce 3D images. Quantitative 3D morphometry using micro-computed tomography (microCT) has been the state of art in technology [96]. This technique is non-destructive and correlates well with conventional histomorphometry [97]. MicroCT allows isotropic resolution (10% MTF, isotropic voxel size 9 µm) (Fig. **6**) which is not achievable in high resolution MR imaging. Thus microCT has been used a reference of standard to validate the high resolution MR (3 Telsa) derived morphometric measures [60]. The significance of the trabecular bone micro-architecture, which adds to the understanding of mechanical properties, has been well illustrated using 3D microtomographic imaging [98, 99]. These studies showed that the parameters of the trabecular bone micro-architecture, in addition to bone density, could add significant variance to account for the elastic modulus and bone strength. The use of microCT has also been validated in other interventional studies. In response to disuse (hindlimb suspension) [100], growth [101], endurance treadmill exercises [102], habitual gait loading [94] and low-level strains at high frequency [103], mechanical interventions as such can induce a specific pattern of change in bone quantity (mass) as well as in bone quality (micro-architecture). Compared to conventional histomorphometry, microCT can show up these changes earlier. This has been evidenced in a recent study in which recombinant human parathyroid hormone (1-34) (teriparatide) improves both cortical and cancellous bone structure [104]. Bone micro-architecture information is therefore an important complement to measures of bone mineral density [91, 105 - 107]. QCT, HR-pQCT and microCT finite element derived biomechanical indices allows non-invasive determination of bone strength (Fig. **7**) [108], monitoring of antiosteoporotic drugs treatment in clinical trials [109, 110], discrimination of men and postmenopausal women with and without fractures [111, 112], respectively.

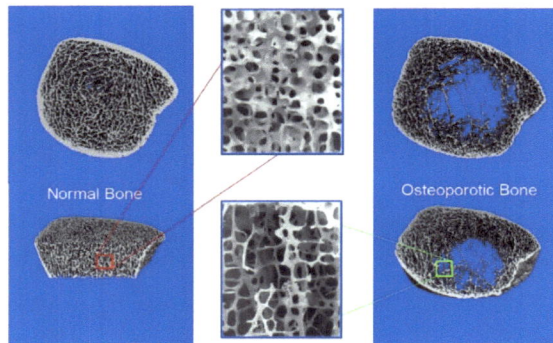

Fig. (6). *In vivo* animal high resolution microCT Courtesy: Bone Quality and Health Centre, Department of Orthopaedics and Traumatology, The Chinese University of Hong Kong).

In Synchrotron radiation (SR)-CT, electrons are accelerated to some GeV by a magnetic field and produce a high photon flux, well collimated, and monochromatic X-ray beams for microscopic imaging. Because of the small divergent angle and monochromaticity of the X-ray beams, it significantly reduces the image distortion and partial volume effect as pertinent in quantitative CT, MicroCT and quantitative MRI. Typical energy resolution is 10^{-4}, which means that the energy spread is less than 5eV [80]. These features render superior contrast resolution at 14-16 bit depth [113, 114] and spatial resolution at 2 μm *in vitro* [115] and 8 μm *in vivo* [116]. High resolutions as such allows the precise demonstration of resorption cavity, trabecular micro-architecture, degree of mineralization [113, 117 - 119].

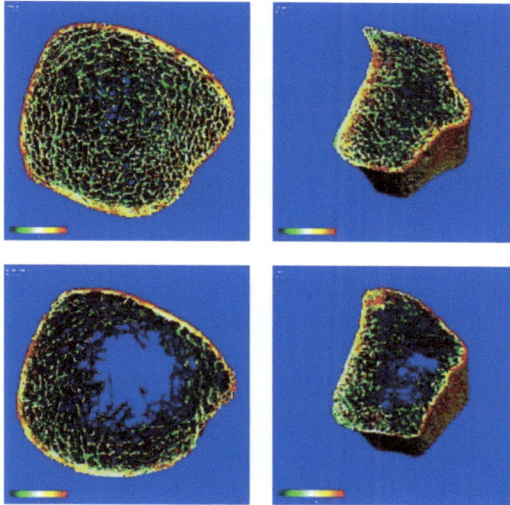

Fig. (7). Finite element analysis of Von Mises stress distribution in distal tibia and radius of normal (upper) verse osteoporotic (lower) female subject (Courtesy: Bone Quality and Health Centre, Department of Orthopaedics and Traumatology, The Chinese University of Hong Kong).

1.2. Imaging of Cortical Bone Micro-Architecture

Measurement of osteon morphometric parameters, including osteon and Haversian dimensions as well as cortical porosities provided the evidence to morphometric differences in human long bone sustained to weight-bearing and non weight-bearing loading [120, 121], in patients with femoral neck fractures [122], and in artiodactyl calcaneus [123] and equine long bone [124, 125] sustained to differential tension/compression loading. Curry studied the cortical porosities and mineral content in 18 species of mammal, bird and reptile, in which over 80% of the total variation in Young's modulus was explained by these two variables [126]. A microCT study by Wachter and August, however, showed that there was no significant improvement in the prediction of cortical bone strength by combining BMD and cortical porosities [127]. Since BMD is a function of both porosities and mineralization, which should explain most of the variance. A study of regional variation in bone status using pQCT by Lai and Qin *et al.* in postmenopausal subjects illustrated that the volumetric BMD at the posterior cortex was significantly higher at 6.5% than the anterior cortex; whereas no significant difference in vBMD was shown between the medial and lateral cortices [93]. However, the anterior cortical wall showed the greatest thickness compared with the other three regions, and was significantly 21.3% greater in thickness than the posterior cortex. It is suggested that geometric adaptation in terms of cortical thickness may be the mechanism to adapt such vBMD differences in response to different strain mode in these regions. MRI also allows quantification of cortical thickness, added that advanced imaging sequence enables the quantification of water content in the minute pores of Haversian system [128, 129]. This circumscribes the limitation of HR-pQCT in demonstration of pore size beyond its resolution limit and provides with a surrogate measure of cortical porosity. Study demonstrated that water content quantification using ultra-short echo time MR imaging in postmenopausal women had 65% greater water content than premenopausal women [130].

1.3. Imaging of Degree of Mineralization

The study by Currey illustrates that there is a considerable range of mineralization measured by ash density ranging from 45% to 58% in non-pathological cortical bone [131]. This range of mineralization results in an even variability of mechanical properties, with the Young modulus of elasticity ranging from 4 to 32 GPa, bending strength from 50 to 300 MPa, and the toughness from 200 to 7000 J/m^2. These mechanical properties are compromised in a bone so as to adapt to the requirement of stiffness, strength and toughness. The same amount of bone mass but with high or lower degree of mineralization corresponds to a high or a low BMD measured either by X-ray absorptiometric and quantitative computed tomographic (QCT) techniques. However, the characteristics of bone mineralization in terms of its degree can be determined by contact microradiography (CMR), backscattered electron (BSE) imaging [9 - 11], ash weight [132], infrared imaging [133 - 135], Raman microspectroscopy [136], histomorphometry with Toluidine Blue (TB) staining [137] (Fig. **6**), Scanning acoustic microscopy (SAM) [138], bench-top microCT with hydroxyapatite phantom calibration [136] and SR-CT [113, 114].

Microradiography is the conventional method for evaluating the degree of mineralization of bone. However, its utility is limited by its volumetric resolution; the errors caused by the projection effect further reduce its accuracy in BMD and histometric analyses. Added to this, calibration between laboratories has yet to be established [9]. Use of ash weight as a measure of degree of mineralization is the gold standard but the method is destructive and does not allow further evaluation of the specimen. Histomorphometry with Toluidine Blue (TB) staining is cost effective. The TB staining intensities in the osteons moderately correlated with the degree of mineralization as measured by CMR using aluminum step wedge as the calibration (r = 0.567) but reliable imaging quantification can be achieved provided that bone matrix is not physiologically fully mineralized [137]. Reflection coefficient as measured by SAM highly correlated with CMR (r = 0.786) [137, 138]. Quantitative BSE imaging has been developed as a tool with high consistency and image resolution [11, 139]. Experimental studies showed that BSE images from canine cortical and trabecular bone had excellent morphologic resolution, accurate bone histomorphometry and the ability to quantify accurately the bone mineralization compared to microradiographic images [140]. It is also advantageous in that it does not have partial volume effect and beam hardening effect as encountered in microCT. These effects do not render the depiction of subtle regional changes in the degree of mineralization. The use of SR-CT with the high intensity, monochromatic X-ray beam provides excellent contrast resolution, which has been applied clinically in the prospective study of the efficacy of antiresorptive drugs on the accretion of bone mineralization and preservation of bone micro-architecture [114, 141, 142]. However, the limited access of SR-CT in worldwide precludes its common use.

The major components of a scanning electron microscope are shown in Fig. **8**. The column is used to generate and focus a narrow beam of electrons upon the specimen mounted in the specimen chamber. The electron gun has a tungsten hairpin filament in which the source of electrons is produced *via* thermionic emission. A series of electromagnetic lens beneath the gun serves to focus and shape the electron beam before it strikes the specimen surface (in case of biological material, like bone, it should be coated with carbon to make it conductive) in a raster scan pattern. The electron beam energy and the electron beam currently can be varied from 300 volts to 30 Kilovolts and from 1 pico-amp to 1 micro-amp, respectively to tailor for the type of examination in progress. The examined specimen is put in a stage inside the chamber. The position of stage can be controlled manually *via* control knob at the front of the stage door to allow for the different views of the specimen.

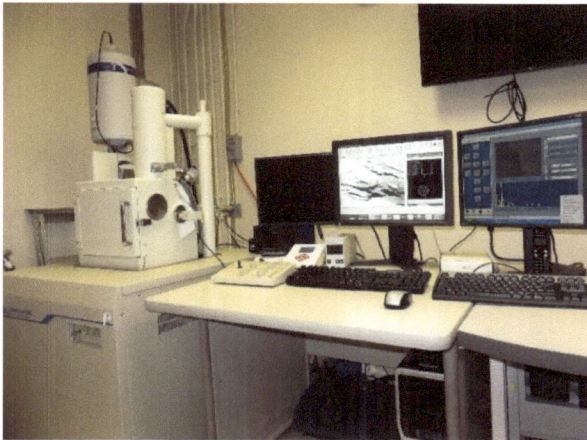

Fig. (8). The major components of a scanning electron microscope.

The operation of the electron optical column and specimen scanning requires a highly vacuum status in the range of 10^{-5} to 10^{-6} torr. The vacuum system is operated by a turbomolecular pump, backed up a rotary pump, is mounted underneath the lower face of the specimen chamber. When the electron beam strikes on the specimen surface, beam specimen interaction gives rise to the emission of Auger electrons, secondary electrons, backscattered electrons, continue and characteristic X-rays from the specimen surface. To study the degree of bone mineralization, a four quadrant back scattered detector (Fig. **9**), is employed to collect the backscattered electrons from the bone specimen. There are several confounding factors in quantitative BSE analysis of bone, which need to be controlled. It is requisite that the incident electron beam maintains the same incident angle and working distance with the specimen [10]. Also, the specimen surface should be highly polished to eliminate the variation of surface topography [143]. Beam current consistency should be monitored using a Faraday cup and a picoampere meter [11]. The amount of backscattered electrons varies directly with the average atomic number of a matter. Accordingly, it allows differentiation of the bone specimen with different degrees of mineralization of the bone matrix as well as the depiction of osteon morphology and porosity (Fig. **10**).

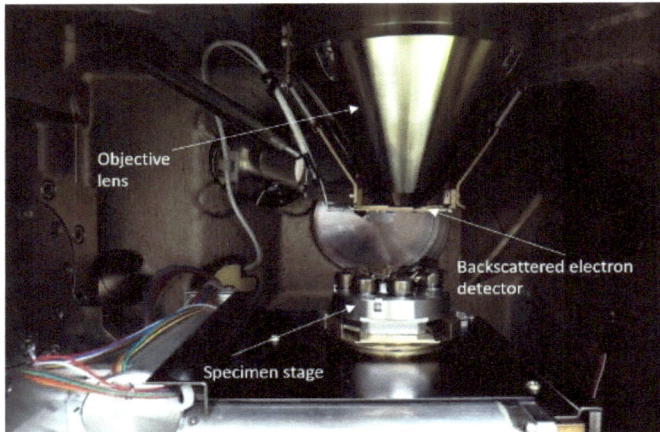

Fig. (9). A four quadrant backscattered detector in situ to collect the backscattered electron signals for BSE imaging.

The efficacy of the degree of mineralization, measured by BSE imaging, in the prediction of bone strength has been validated in experimental studies using standardized machined bovine bone samples [144, 145], in baboon [146] and human studies prescribed with anti-resorptive Alendronate [147] and anabolic teriparatide [133] and in comparing the efficacy weight bearing and non-weight bearing exercise interventions [148]. The study by Follet and Boivin *et al.* using human cadaveric calcanei supported the findings that the increase in bone strength was augmented by degree of mineralization within the physiological range without necessary changes of bone matrix volume and micro-architecture [149].

Similar findings were also observed in ovariectomized baboons treated with alendronate [146], in postmenopausal osteoporotic patients treated with alendronate [147], in postmenopausal osteoporotic patients treated with risedronate [114, 142].

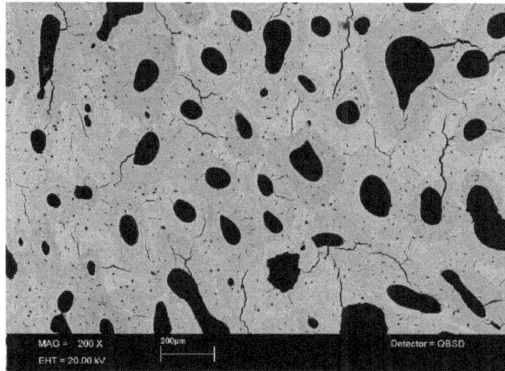

Fig. (10). Micrograph of backscattered electron imaging of cadaveric tibial cortex showing different degree of mineralization.

1.4. Imaging of Collagen Fibre Orientation

The orientation of collagen fibres can be demonstrated using polarized light microscopy [144, 150 - 154] (Fig. **11**). The use of circularly polarized light, as opposed to linearly polarized light, to study collagen fibre orientation has been validated in terms of its better correlation with mechanical properties. Also, the quantification of fibre orientation using circularly polarized light microscopy is superior in that it is independent of the orientation of a specimen in the field of view and is without maltase cross artefacts [152].

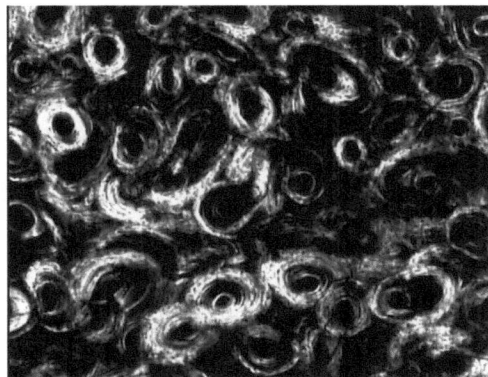

Fig. (11). Circularly polarized light micrograph showing an undecalcifed section of cortical bone from a human tibia.

The principle of circularly polarized light microscopy has been described in details [12]. The set-up of the microscopic imaging is shown in Fig. **12**. First, the polarizer and analyser are set with its optical transmission axis 90 degree to each other. As such it creates background extinction. A quarter wave plate is inserted between the polarizer and the bone specimen whereas another is placed between the bone specimen and the analyser. This arrangement of quarter wave plates aims to restore the background extinction. The unpolarized light source after passing through the polarizer becomes linearly polarized. That is vibration of the light wave is only confined in one plane that coincides with the optical transmission axis of the polarizer. The plane polarized light incident on the quarter wave plate resolves into two orthogonal wave components (birefringent effect) with equal magnitude but propagating with a phase difference of a quarter wavelength ($\lambda/4$). This results in a circularly polarized light (CPL) wave with its electric vector rotating in 360 degrees. The CPL will refract in the bone specimen such that its birefringent effect allows transmission of peak light intensities on condition that the collagen fibres lying parallel (transverse orientation) with plane of bone section. The emerging CPL from the bone specimen incident on the quarter wave plate will then be converted into linearly polarized light and aligns with the transmission axis of the analyser.

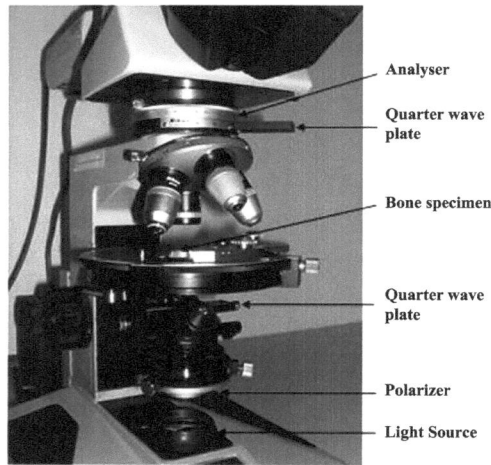

Fig. (12). Circularly polarized light microscopy set up.

Preferred longitudinal collagen fibre orientation (CFO) has been shown in the tension cortex, whereas a more transverse-to-oblique direction is seen in the compression cortex of the equine radius [151, 155] and in human upper and lower limb shafts [150, 156]. Thus the use of CPL in the demonstration of CFO may add evidence to the regional differences in cortical cBMD of long bone shaft [93]. The CFO quantified as the predominant longitudinal direction explained the greatest percentage of variance in the total amount of energy absorbed in the ultimate tensile stress using equine third metacarpals at mid-diaphysis [157]. It was also the best predictor of tensile strength [144] and bending elastic modulus and ultimate stress using bovine cortical bone [145].

1.5. Imaging of Microdamage

Microdamage in the bones can result from cyclic loading, within their elastic limits, at sufficient intensity [158]. *In vivo* linear microcracks in human ribs have been demonstrated at light microscopic level using validated en bloc staining method with basic fuchsin, which allows separation of artifactual and non-artifactual cracks [13]. In both men and women after the age of 40, there is an exponential increase in linear crack density in the femoral cortex, with the damage occurs about twice as fast in women as in men [159]. However, such age-related increase and accumulation in microdamage with repair failure has yet been shown equivocally to cause bone fragility, but rather the positive feedback mechanism between the microdamage and remodelling may accelerate failure [160]. There was no age-dependent accumulation of diffuse microdamage, as identified by validated confocal microscopy, in male or female vertebral trabecular bone [161]. It is argued that the spine has a high turnover rate and the damage accumulation. The results may not be generalized to the appendicular sites.

The accumulation of microdamage, in response to cyclic loading, associates with the decline in mechanical properties is well supported by numerous studies [160, 162 - 166]. Strain mode was shown to relate to the differences in microdamage morphology. It was demonstrated that in-vitro canine femur subjected to four-point cyclic bending had got linear microcrack accumulation more rapidly in tensile cortices, but the crack length was greater in compression cortex. The rapid accumulation of microdamage would at the same time initiate a greater remodelling rate [160, 167]. This may result in lower bone mineral density in the tension cortices as compared to the compression cortex. It was illustrated that the volumetric BMD (vBMD) of the posterior compression cortex, in human distal tibia under habitual gait loading, was a significant 6.5% higher than that of the anterior tension cortex ($P<0.001$) [93]. Recent study in human cortical bone shows that microdamage in terms of numerical density and crack length are significantly greater in interstitial bone parallel with a significantly lower osteocyte lacunae density when compared to the osteonal bone [168]. Investigation of the microdamage morphology between the cortices subject to differential strain/mode may provide further understanding of the regional vBMD differences.

2. SUMMARY

Material and structural properties are determinants of bone strength. Synergised use of multi-modality imaging methods including quantitative ultrasound, high resolution magnetic resonance imaging and computed tomography, polarised light microscopy, backscattered electron imaging and advanced image processing techniques offers important information of bone status beyond bone mineral density. This has deciphered insights into understanding the effects of pharmaceutical and biophysical interventions on bone responses and the interplay among the determinants of bone strength.

CONFLICT OF INTEREST

The author(s) confirm that this chapter contents have no conflict of interest.

ACKNOWLEDGEMENTS

Declared none

REFERENCES

[1]   Frost HM. Bone "mass" and the "mechanostat": a proposal. Anat Rec 1987; 219(1): 1-9.
        [http://dx.doi.org/10.1002/ar.1092190104] [PMID: 3688455]

[2]   Jee WSS. Principles in bone physiology. J Musculoskelet Neuronal Interact 2000; 1(1): 11-3.
        [PMID: 15758518]

[3]   Genant HK, Gordon C, Jiang Y, *et al.* Advanced imaging of the macrostructure and microstructure of
        bone. Horm Res 2000; 54 (Suppl. 1): 24-30.
        [http://dx.doi.org/10.1159/000063444] [PMID: 11146376]

[4]   Genant HK, Engelke K, Fuerst T, *et al.* Noninvasive assessment of bone mineral and structure: state of
        the art. J Bone Miner Res 1996; 11(6): 707-30.
        [http://dx.doi.org/10.1002/jbmr.5650110602] [PMID: 8725168]

[5]   Genant HK, Lang TF, Engelke K, *et al.* Advances in the noninvasive assessment of bone density,
        quality, and structure. Calcif Tissue Int 1996; 59(7) (Suppl. 1): S10-5.
        [http://dx.doi.org/10.1007/s002239900169] [PMID: 8974723]

[6]   Genant HK, Gordon C, Jiang Y, Lang TF, Link TM, Majumdar S. Advanced imaging of bone macro
        and micro structure. Bone 1999; 25(1): 149-52.
        [http://dx.doi.org/10.1016/S8756-3282(99)00109-X] [PMID: 10423042]

[7]   Van Kuijk C, Genant HK. Bone Densitometry Orthopedic Imaging: Techniques and Applications.
        Springer-Verlag: Berline 1998; pp. 143-52.
        [http://dx.doi.org/10.1007/978-3-642-60295-5_9]

[8]   Wong DM, Sartoris DJ. Noninvasive Methods for Assessment of Bone Density, Architecture, and
        Biomechanical Properties: Fundamental Concepts.Osteoporosis: Diagnosis and Treatment. New York:
        M. Dekker 1996; pp. 201-32.

[9]   Bloebaum RD, Skedros JG, Vajda EG, Bachus KN, Constantz BR. Determining mineral content
        variations in bone using backscattered electron imaging. Bone 1997; 20(5): 485-90.
        [http://dx.doi.org/10.1016/S8756-3282(97)00015-X] [PMID: 9145247]

[10]   Bloebaum RD, Bachus KN, Boyce TM. Backscattered electron imaging: the role in calcified tissue and implant analysis. J Biomater Appl 1990; 5(1): 56-85.
[PMID: 2200867]

[11]   Roschger P, Fratzl P, Eschberger J, Klaushofer K. Validation of quantitative backscattered electron imaging for the measurement of mineral density distribution in human bone biopsies. Bone 1998; 23(4): 319-26.
[http://dx.doi.org/10.1016/S8756-3282(98)00112-4] [PMID: 9763143]

[12]   Bromage TG, Goldman HM, McFarlin SC, Warshaw J, Boyde A, Riggs CM. Circularly polarized light standards for investigations of collagen fiber orientation in bone. Anat Rec B New Anat 2003; 274(1): 157-68.
[http://dx.doi.org/10.1002/ar.b.10031] [PMID: 12964206]

[13]   Burr DB, Stafford T. Validity of the bulk-staining technique to separate artifactual from *in vivo* bone microdamage. Clin Orthop Relat Res 1990; (260): 305-8.
[PMID: 1699696]

[14]   Martin RB. Fatigue microdamage as an essential element of bone mechanics and biology. Calcif Tissue Int 2003; 73(2): 101-7.
[http://dx.doi.org/10.1007/s00223-002-1059-9] [PMID: 14565590]

[15]   Genant HK, Majumdar S. High-resolution magnetic resonance imaging of trabecular bone structure. Osteoporos Int 1997; 7 (Suppl. 3): S135-9.
[http://dx.doi.org/10.1007/BF03194359] [PMID: 9536319]

[16]   Majumdar S, Kothari M, Augat P, *et al.* High-resolution magnetic resonance imaging: three-dimensional trabecular bone architecture and biomechanical properties. Bone 1998; 22(5): 445-54.
[http://dx.doi.org/10.1016/S8756-3282(98)00030-1] [PMID: 9600777]

[17]   Jiang Y, Zhao J, White DL, Genant HK. Micro CT and Micro MR imaging of 3D architecture of animal skeleton. J Musculoskelet Neuronal Interact 2000; 1(1): 45-51.
[PMID: 15758525]

[18]   Link TM, Bauer JS. Imaging of trabecular bone structure. Semin Musculoskelet Radiol 2002; 6(3): 253-61.
[http://dx.doi.org/10.1055/s-2002-36723] [PMID: 12541203]

[19]   Link TM. Structure Analysis using High-Resolution Imaging Techniques. Radiology of Osteoporosis. Berlin: Springer-Verlag 2003; pp. 153-64.
[http://dx.doi.org/10.1007/978-3-662-05235-8_12]

[20]   Ito M, *et al.* Multi-detector-Row CT Imaging of Verterbral Microstructure for Evaluation of Fracture Risk. Bone 2005; 36: s324-5.

[21]   Link TM, Majumdar S, Lin JC, *et al.* A comparative study of trabecular bone properties in the spine and femur using high resolution MRI and CT. J Bone Miner Res 1998; 13(1): 122-32.
[http://dx.doi.org/10.1359/jbmr.1998.13.1.122] [PMID: 9443798]

[22]   Link TM, Vieth V, Matheis J, *et al.* Bone structure of the distal radius and the calcaneus *vs.* BMD of the spine and proximal femur in the prediction of osteoporotic spine fractures. Eur Radiol 2002; 12(2): 401-8.
[http://dx.doi.org/10.1007/s003300101127] [PMID: 11870442]

[23]   Link TM, Vieth V, Stehling C, *et al.* High-resolution MRI *vs.* multislice spiral CT: which technique depicts the trabecular bone structure best? Eur Radiol 2003; 13(4): 663-71.
[PMID: 12664101]

[24]   Majumdar S, Link TM, Augat P, *et al.* Trabecular bone architecture in the distal radius using magnetic resonance imaging in subjects with fractures of the proximal femur. Osteoporos Int 1999; 10(3): 231-9.
[http://dx.doi.org/10.1007/s001980050221] [PMID: 10525716]

[25]   Singh M, Nagrath AR, Maini PS. Changes in trabecular pattern of the upper end of the femur as an index of osteoporosis. J Bone Joint Surg Am 1970; 52(3): 457-67.
[http://dx.doi.org/10.2106/00004623-197052030-00005] [PMID: 5425640]

[26]   Chen J, Zheng B, Chang YH, Shaw CC, Towers JD, Gur D. Fractal analysis of trabecular patterns in projection radiographs. An assessment. Invest Radiol 1994; 29(6): 624-9.
[http://dx.doi.org/10.1097/00004424-199406000-00005] [PMID: 8088971]

[27]   Veenland JF, Grashius JL, van der Meer F, Beckers AL, Gelsema ES. Estimation of fractal dimension in radiographs. Med Phys 1996; 23(4): 585-94.
[http://dx.doi.org/10.1118/1.597816] [PMID: 8860906]

[28]   Lin JC, Grampp S, Link T, *et al.* Fractal analysis of proximal femur radiographs: correlation with biomechanical properties and bone mineral density. Osteoporos Int 1999; 9(6): 516-24.
[http://dx.doi.org/10.1007/s001980050179] [PMID: 10624459]

[29]   Langton CM, Palmer SB, Porter RW. The measurement of broadband ultrasonic attenuation in cancellous bone. Eng Med 1984; 13(2): 89-91.
[http://dx.doi.org/10.1243/EMED_JOUR_1984_013_022_02] [PMID: 6540216]

[30]   Njeh CF, Boivin CM, Langton CM. The role of ultrasound in the assessment of osteoporosis: a review. Osteoporos Int 1997; 7(1): 7-22.
[http://dx.doi.org/10.1007/BF01623454] [PMID: 9102067]

[31]   Stewart A, Reid DM. Quantitative ultrasound in osteoporosis. Semin Musculoskelet Radiol 2002; 6(3): 229-32.
[http://dx.doi.org/10.1055/s-2002-36720] [PMID: 12541200]

[32]   Kaufman JJ, Einhorn TA. Ultrasound assessment of bone. J Bone Miner Res 1993; 8(5): 517-25.
[http://dx.doi.org/10.1002/jbmr.5650080502] [PMID: 8511979]

[33]   Hans D, Schott AM, Meunier PJ. Ultrasonic assessment of bone: a review. Eur J Med 1993; 2(3): 157-63.
[PMID: 8261057]

[34]   Hans D, Wu C, Njeh CF, *et al.* Ultrasound velocity of trabecular cubes reflects mainly bone density and elasticity. Calcif Tissue Int 1999; 64(1): 18-23.
[http://dx.doi.org/10.1007/s002239900572] [PMID: 9868278]

[35]   Hodgskinson R, Njeh CF, Currey JD, Langton CM. The ability of ultrasound velocity to predict the stiffness of cancellous bone in vitro. Bone 1997; 21(2): 183-90.
[http://dx.doi.org/10.1016/S8756-3282(97)00098-7] [PMID: 9267694]

[36]   Hans D, *et al.* Quantitative Ultrasound for Assessing Bone Properties. Bone Densitometry and Osteoporosis. Berlin: Springer 1998; pp. 378-405.
[http://dx.doi.org/10.1007/978-3-642-80440-3_19]

[37]   Tromp AM, Smit JH, Deeg DJ, Lips P. Quantitative ultrasound measurements of the tibia and calcaneus in comparison with DXA measurements at various skeletal sites. Osteoporos Int 1999; 9(3): 230-5.
[http://dx.doi.org/10.1007/s001980050142] [PMID: 10450412]

[38]   Yeap SS, Pearson D, Cawte SA, Hosking DJ. The relationship between bone mineral density and ultrasound in postmenopausal and osteoporotic women. Osteoporos Int 1998; 8(2): 141-6.
[http://dx.doi.org/10.1007/BF02672510] [PMID: 9666937]

[39]   Hung VW, Qin L, Au SK, *et al.* Correlations of calcaneal QUS with pQCT measurements at distal tibia and non-weight-bearing distal radius. J Bone Miner Metab 2004; 22(5): 486-90.
[http://dx.doi.org/10.1007/s00774-004-0511-5] [PMID: 15316870]

[40]   Bauer DC, Glüer CC, Cauley JA, *et al.* Broadband ultrasound attenuation predicts fractures strongly and independently of densitometry in older women. A prospective study. Arch Intern Med 1997;

157(6): 629-34. [see comments].
[http://dx.doi.org/10.1001/archinte.1997.00440270067006] [PMID: 9080917]

[41] Hans D, Dargent-Molina P, Schott AM, *et al.* Ultrasonographic heel measurements to predict hip fracture in elderly women: the EPIDOS prospective study. Lancet 1996; 348(9026): 511-4.
[http://dx.doi.org/10.1016/S0140-6736(95)11456-4] [PMID: 8757153]

[42] Kim CH, Kim YI, Choi CS, *et al.* Prevalence and risk factors of low quantitative ultrasound values of calcaneus in Korean elderly women. Ultrasound Med Biol 2000; 26(1): 35-40.
[http://dx.doi.org/10.1016/S0301-5629(99)00126-X] [PMID: 10687790]

[43] Baran DT. Quantitative ultrasound: a technique to target women with low bone mass for preventive therapy. Am J Med 1995; 98(2A): 48S-51S.
[http://dx.doi.org/10.1016/S0002-9343(05)80046-4] [PMID: 7709935]

[44] Glüer CC, Hans D. How to use ultrasound for risk assessment: a need for defining strategies. Osteoporos Int 1999; 9(3): 193-5. [editorial].
[http://dx.doi.org/10.1007/s001980050135] [PMID: 10450405]

[45] Glüer CC, Eastell R, Reid DM, *et al.* Association of five quantitative ultrasound devices and bone densitometry with osteoporotic vertebral fractures in a population-based sample: the OPUS Study. J Bone Miner Res 2004; 19(5): 782-93.
[http://dx.doi.org/10.1359/jbmr.040304] [PMID: 15068502]

[46] Skerry TM. Mechanical loading and bone: what sort of exercise is beneficial to the skeleton? Bone 1997; 20(3): 179-81.
[http://dx.doi.org/10.1016/S8756-3282(96)00387-0] [PMID: 9071466]

[47] Wolff I, van Croonenborg JJ, Kemper HC, Kostense PJ, Twisk JW. The effect of exercise training programs on bone mass: a meta-analysis of published controlled trials in pre- and postmenopausal women. Osteoporos Int 1999; 9(1): 1-12.
[http://dx.doi.org/10.1007/s001980050109] [PMID: 10367023]

[48] Kohrt WM, Ehsani AA, Birge SJ Jr. Effects of exercise involving predominantly either joint-reaction or ground-reaction forces on bone mineral density in older women. J Bone Miner Res 1997; 12(8): 1253-61.
[http://dx.doi.org/10.1359/jbmr.1997.12.8.1253] [PMID: 9258756]

[49] Judex S, Zernicke RF. High-impact exercise and growing bone: relation between high strain rates and enhanced bone formation. J Appl Physiol 2000; 88(6): 2183-91.
[http://dx.doi.org/10.1152/jappl.2000.88.6.2183] [PMID: 10846034]

[50] Simkin A, Ayalon J, Leichter I. Increased trabecular bone density due to bone-loading exercises in postmenopausal osteoporotic women. Calcif Tissue Int 1987; 40(2): 59-63.
[http://dx.doi.org/10.1007/BF02555706] [PMID: 3105835]

[51] Yung PS, Lai YM, Tung PY, *et al.* Effects of weight bearing and non-weight bearing exercises on bone properties using calcaneal quantitative ultrasound. Br J Sports Med 2005; 39(8): 547-51.
[http://dx.doi.org/10.1136/bjsm.2004.014621] [PMID: 16046341]

[52] Falk B, Bronshtein Z, Zigel L, Constantini NW, Eliakim A. Quantitative ultrasound of the tibia and radius in prepubertal and early-pubertal female athletes. Arch Pediatr Adolesc Med 2003; 157(2): 139-43.
[http://dx.doi.org/10.1001/archpedi.157.2.139] [PMID: 12580682]

[53] Graham DT. Principles of Radiological Physics. 3rd ed. New York: Churchhill Livingstone 1996; pp. 581-4.

[54] Grampp S, Majumdar S, Jergas M, Lang P, Gies A, Genant HK. MRI of bone marrow in the distal radius: *in vivo* precision of effective transverse relaxation times. Eur Radiol 1995; 5(1): 43-8.
[http://dx.doi.org/10.1007/BF00178080] [PMID: 11539927]

[55] Davis CA, Genant HK, Dunham JS. The effects of bone on proton NMR relaxation times of

surrounding liquids. Invest Radiol 1986; 21(6): 472-7.
[http://dx.doi.org/10.1097/00004424-198606000-00005] [PMID: 3721804]

[56] Rosenthal H, Thulborn KR, Rosenthal DI, Kim SH, Rosen BR. Magnetic susceptibility effects of trabecular bone on magnetic resonance imaging of bone marrow. Invest Radiol 1990; 25(2): 173-8.
[http://dx.doi.org/10.1097/00004424-199002000-00013] [PMID: 2312252]

[57] Majumdar S, Genant HK. *In vivo* relationship between marrow T2* and trabecular bone density determined with a chemical shift-selective asymmetric spin-echo sequence. J Magn Reson Imaging 1992; 2(2): 209-19.
[http://dx.doi.org/10.1002/jmri.1880020215] [PMID: 1562773]

[58] Lai YM, Qin L, Hung VW, *et al.* Trabecular bone status in ultradistal tibia under habitual gait loading: a pQCT study in postmenopausal women. J Clin Densitom 2006; 9(2): 175-83.
[http://dx.doi.org/10.1016/j.jocd.2005.11.006] [PMID: 16785078]

[59] Majumdar S, Newitt D, Jergas M, *et al.* Evaluation of technical factors affecting the quantification of trabecular bone structure using magnetic resonance imaging. Bone 1995; 17(4): 417-30.
[http://dx.doi.org/10.1016/S8756-3282(95)00263-4] [PMID: 8573417]

[60] Sell CA, Masi JN, Burghardt A, Newitt D, Link TM, Majumdar S. Quantification of trabecular bone structure using magnetic resonance imaging at 3 Tesla--calibration studies using microcomputed tomography as a standard of reference. Calcif Tissue Int 2005; 76(5): 355-64.
[http://dx.doi.org/10.1007/s00223-004-0111-3] [PMID: 15868282]

[61] Link TM, Majumdar S, Augat P, *et al.* *In vivo* high resolution MRI of the calcaneus: differences in trabecular structure in osteoporosis patients. J Bone Miner Res 1998; 13(7): 1175-82.
[http://dx.doi.org/10.1359/jbmr.1998.13.7.1175] [PMID: 9661082]

[62] Weber MH, Sharp JC, Latta P, Sramek M, Hassard HT, Orr FW. Magnetic resonance imaging of trabecular and cortical bone in mice: comparison of high resolution *in vivo* and ex vivo MR images with corresponding histology. Eur J Radiol 2005; 53(1): 96-102.
[http://dx.doi.org/10.1016/j.ejrad.2004.02.009] [PMID: 15607859]

[63] Boehm HF, Raeth C, Monetti RA, *et al.* Local 3D scaling properties for the analysis of trabecular bone extracted from high-resolution magnetic resonance imaging of human trabecular bone: comparison with bone mineral density in the prediction of biomechanical strength in vitro. Invest Radiol 2003; 38(5): 269-80.
[http://dx.doi.org/10.1097/01.RLI.0000064782.94757.0f] [PMID: 12750616]

[64] Jergas MD, Majumdar S, Keyak JH, *et al.* Relationships between young modulus of elasticity, ash density, and MRI derived effective transverse relaxation T2* in tibial specimens. J Comput Assist Tomogr 1995; 19(3): 472-9.
[http://dx.doi.org/10.1097/00004728-199505000-00024] [PMID: 7790561]

[65] Majumdar S, Newitt D, Mathur A, *et al.* Magnetic resonance imaging of trabecular bone structure in the distal radius: relationship with X-ray tomographic microscopy and biomechanics. Osteoporos Int 1996; 6(5): 376-85.
[http://dx.doi.org/10.1007/BF01623011] [PMID: 8931032]

[66] Borah B, Dufresne TE, Cockman MD, *et al.* Evaluation of changes in trabecular bone architecture and mechanical properties of minipig vertebrae by three-dimensional magnetic resonance microimaging and finite element modeling. J Bone Miner Res 2000; 15(9): 1786-97.
[http://dx.doi.org/10.1359/jbmr.2000.15.9.1786] [PMID: 10976998]

[67] Beuf O, Newitt DC, Mosekilde L, Majumdar S. Trabecular structure assessment in lumbar vertebrae specimens using quantitative magnetic resonance imaging and relationship with mechanical competence. J Bone Miner Res 2001; 16(8): 1511-9.
[http://dx.doi.org/10.1359/jbmr.2001.16.8.1511] [PMID: 11499874]

[68] Wehrli FW, Hwang SN, Ma J, Song HK, Ford JC, Haddad JG. Cancellous bone volume and structure in the forearm: noninvasive assessment with MR microimaging and image processing. Radiology

1998; 206(2): 347-57.
[http://dx.doi.org/10.1148/radiology.206.2.9457185] [PMID: 9457185]

[69]　Wehrli FW, Gomberg BR, Saha PK, Song HK, Hwang SN, Snyder PJ. Digital topological analysis of *in vivo* magnetic resonance microimages of trabecular bone reveals structural implications of osteoporosis. J Bone Miner Res 2001; 16(8): 1520-31.
[http://dx.doi.org/10.1359/jbmr.2001.16.8.1520] [PMID: 11499875]

[70]　Wehrli FW, Saha PK, Gomberg BR, *et al.* Role of magnetic resonance for assessing structure and function of trabecular bone. Top Magn Reson Imaging 2002; 13(5): 335-55.
[http://dx.doi.org/10.1097/00002142-200210000-00005] [PMID: 12464746]

[71]　Bernard CP, Liney GP, Manton DJ, Turnbull LW, Langton CM. Comparison of fat quantification methods: a phantom study at 3.0T. J Magn Reson Imaging 2008; 27(1): 192-7.
[http://dx.doi.org/10.1002/jmri.21201] [PMID: 18064714]

[72]　Schellinger D, Lin CS, Hatipoglu HG, Fertikh D. Potential value of vertebral proton MR spectroscopy in determining bone weakness. AJNR Am J Neuroradiol 2001; 22(8): 1620-7.
[PMID: 11559519]

[73]　Li G, Xu Z, Gu H, *et al.* Comparison of chemical shift-encoded water-fat MRI and MR spectroscopy in quantification of marrow fat in postmenopausal females. J Magn Reson Imaging 2016.
[PMID: 27341545]

[74]　Justesen J, Stenderup K, Ebbesen EN, Mosekilde L, Steiniche T, Kassem M. Adipocyte tissue volume in bone marrow is increased with aging and in patients with osteoporosis. Biogerontology 2001; 2(3): 165-71.
[http://dx.doi.org/10.1023/A:1011513223894] [PMID: 11708718]

[75]　Yeung DK, Griffith JF, Antonio GE, Lee FK, Woo J, Leung PC. Osteoporosis is associated with increased marrow fat content and decreased marrow fat unsaturation: a proton MR spectroscopy study. J Magn Reson Imaging 2005; 22(2): 279-85.
[http://dx.doi.org/10.1002/jmri.20367] [PMID: 16028245]

[76]　Griffith JF, Yeung DK, Antonio GE, *et al.* Vertebral marrow fat content and diffusion and perfusion indexes in women with varying bone density: MR evaluation. Radiology 2006; 241(3): 831-8.
[http://dx.doi.org/10.1148/radiol.2413051858] [PMID: 17053202]

[77]　Griffith JF, Yeung DK, Tsang PH, *et al.* Compromised bone marrow perfusion in osteoporosis. J Bone Miner Res 2008; 23(7): 1068-75.
[http://dx.doi.org/10.1359/jbmr.080233] [PMID: 18302498]

[78]　Griffith JF, Yeung DK, Antonio GE, *et al.* Vertebral bone mineral density, marrow perfusion, and fat content in healthy men and men with osteoporosis: dynamic contrast-enhanced MR imaging and MR spectroscopy. Radiology 2005; 236(3): 945-51.
[http://dx.doi.org/10.1148/radiol.2363041425] [PMID: 16055699]

[79]　Romans LE. Introduction to computed tomography. Baltimore: Williams & Wilkins 1995.

[80]　Ruegsegger P. Imaging of Bone Structure. Bone mechanics handbook. Boca Raton, Fla.: CRC Press 2001; pp. 9-1-9-24.

[81]　Müller R, Hildebrand T, Rüegsegger P. Non-invasive bone biopsy: a new method to analyse and display the three-dimensional structure of trabecular bone. Phys Med Biol 1994; 39(1): 145-64.
[http://dx.doi.org/10.1088/0031-9155/39/1/009] [PMID: 7651993]

[82]　Ruegsegger P. The use of peripherial QCT in the evaluation of bone remodelling. Endocrinologist 1994; 4: 167-76.
[http://dx.doi.org/10.1097/00019616-199405000-00004]

[83]　Qin L, Au S, Choy W, *et al.* Regular Tai Chi Chuan exercise may retard bone loss in postmenopausal women: A case-control study. Arch Phys Med Rehabil 2002; 83(10): 1355-9.
[http://dx.doi.org/10.1053/apmr.2002.35098] [PMID: 12370867]

[84]   Qin L, Au SK, Leung PC, *et al.* Baseline BMD and Bone Loss at Distal Radius Measured by pQCT in Peri- and Postmenopausal Hong Kong Chinese Women. Osteoporos Int 2002; 13(12): 962-70. [http://dx.doi.org/10.1007/s001980200134] [PMID: 12459939]

[85]   Chan K, Qin L, Lau M, *et al.* A randomized, prospective study of the effects of Tai Chi Chun exercise on bone mineral density in postmenopausal women. Arch Phys Med Rehabil 2004; 85(5): 717-22. [http://dx.doi.org/10.1016/j.apmr.2003.08.091] [PMID: 15129394]

[86]   Seeram E. Image Quality.Computed tomography: physical principles, clinical applications, and quality control. Philadelphia: W.B. Saunders 2001.

[87]   Augat P, Fuerst T, Genant HK. Quantitative bone mineral assessment at the forearm: a review. Osteoporos Int 1998; 8(4): 299-310. [http://dx.doi.org/10.1007/s001980050068] [PMID: 10024899]

[88]   Qin L, Au SK, Chan KM, *et al.* Peripheral volumetric bone mineral density in pre- and postmenopausal Chinese women in Hong Kong. Calcif Tissue Int 2000; 67(1): 29-36. [http://dx.doi.org/10.1007/s00223001092] [PMID: 10908409]

[89]   Chan KM, *et al.* Using peripheral quantitative computed tomography (pQCT) to monitor the effect of one-year Tai-Chi on bone loss in postmenopausal women. Osteoporos Int 2000; 11 (Suppl. 3): s5.

[90]   Hassager C, Jensen SB, Gotfredsen A, Christiansen C. The impact of measurement errors on the diagnostic value of bone mass measurements: theoretical considerations. Osteoporos Int 1991; 1(4): 250-6. [http://dx.doi.org/10.1007/BF03187470] [PMID: 1790412]

[91]   Jiang Y, Zhao J, Augat P, *et al.* Trabecular bone mineral and calculated structure of human bone specimens scanned by peripheral quantitative computed tomography: relation to biomechanical properties. J Bone Miner Res 1998; 13(11): 1783-90. [http://dx.doi.org/10.1359/jbmr.1998.13.11.1783] [PMID: 9797489]

[92]   Wachter NJ, Augat P, Mentzel M, *et al.* Predictive value of bone mineral density and morphology determined by peripheral quantitative computed tomography for cancellous bone strength of the proximal femur. Bone 2001; 28(1): 133-9. [http://dx.doi.org/10.1016/S8756-3282(00)00455-5] [PMID: 11165955]

[93]   Lai YM, Qin L, Hung VW, Chan KM. Regional differences in cortical bone mineral density in the weight-bearing long bone shaft--a pQCT study. Bone 2005; 36(3): 465-71. [http://dx.doi.org/10.1016/j.bone.2004.11.005] [PMID: 15777653]

[94]   Lai YM, Qin L, Yeung HY, Lee KK, Chan KM. Regional differences in trabecular BMD and micro-architecture of weight-bearing bone under habitual gait loading--a pQCT and microCT study in human cadavers. Bone 2005; 37(2): 274-82. [http://dx.doi.org/10.1016/j.bone.2005.04.025] [PMID: 15961358]

[95]   Dambacher M, *et al.* XTREMECT" A New Dimension in Bone Micro Architecture Evaluation *in vivo* in Humans. Bone 2005; 36: s324.

[96]   Rüegsegger P, Koller B, Müller R. A microtomographic system for the nondestructive evaluation of bone architecture. Calcif Tissue Int 1996; 58(1): 24-9. [http://dx.doi.org/10.1007/BF02509542] [PMID: 8825235]

[97]   Müller R, Van Campenhout H, Van Damme B, *et al.* Morphometric analysis of human bone biopsies: a quantitative structural comparison of histological sections and micro-computed tomography. Bone 1998; 23(1): 59-66. [http://dx.doi.org/10.1016/S8756-3282(98)00068-4] [PMID: 9662131]

[98]   Ulrich D, van Rietbergen B, Laib A, Rüegsegger P. The ability of three-dimensional structural indices to reflect mechanical aspects of trabecular bone. Bone 1999; 25(1): 55-60. [http://dx.doi.org/10.1016/S8756-3282(99)00098-8] [PMID: 10423022]

[99]   Goldstein SA, Goulet R, McCubbrey D. Measurement and significance of three-dimensional architecture to the mechanical integrity of trabecular bone. Calcif Tissue Int 1993; 53(Suppl 1): S127-32. discussion S132-3
[http://dx.doi.org/10.1007/BF01673421]

[100]   David V, Laroche N, Boudignon B, *et al.* Noninvasive *in vivo* monitoring of bone architecture alterations in hindlimb-unloaded female rats using novel three-dimensional microcomputed tomography. J Bone Miner Res 2003; 18(9): 1622-31.
[http://dx.doi.org/10.1359/jbmr.2003.18.9.1622] [PMID: 12968671]

[101]   Tanck E, Homminga J, van Lenthe GH, Huiskes R. Increase in bone volume fraction precedes architectural adaptation in growing bone. Bone 2001; 28(6): 650-4.
[http://dx.doi.org/10.1016/S8756-3282(01)00464-1] [PMID: 11425654]

[102]   Joo YI, Sone T, Fukunaga M, Lim SG, Onodera S. Effects of endurance exercise on three-dimensional trabecular bone microarchitecture in young growing rats. Bone 2003; 33(4): 485-93.
[http://dx.doi.org/10.1016/S8756-3282(03)00212-6] [PMID: 14555251]

[103]   Rubin C, Turner AS, Müller R, *et al.* Quantity and quality of trabecular bone in the femur are enhanced by a strongly anabolic, noninvasive mechanical intervention. J Bone Miner Res 2002; 17(2): 349-57.
[http://dx.doi.org/10.1359/jbmr.2002.17.2.349] [PMID: 11811566]

[104]   Jiang Y, Zhao JJ, Mitlak BH, Wang O, Genant HK, Eriksen EF. Recombinant human parathyroid hormone (1-34) [teriparatide] improves both cortical and cancellous bone structure. J Bone Miner Res 2003; 18(11): 1932-41.
[http://dx.doi.org/10.1359/jbmr.2003.18.11.1932] [PMID: 14606504]

[105]   Delmas PD. Do we need to change the WHO definition of osteoporosis? Osteoporos Int 2000; 11(3): 189-91.
[http://dx.doi.org/10.1007/s001980050280] [PMID: 10824233]

[106]   Link TM, Majumdar S, Grampp S, *et al.* Imaging of trabecular bone structure in osteoporosis. Eur Radiol 1999; 9(9): 1781-8.
[http://dx.doi.org/10.1007/s003300050922] [PMID: 10602950]

[107]   Dempster DW. The contribution of trabecular architecture to cancellous bone quality. J Bone Miner Res 2000; 15(1): 20-3.
[http://dx.doi.org/10.1359/jbmr.2000.15.1.20] [PMID: 10646110]

[108]   van Rietbergen B. Micro-FE analyses of bone: state of the art. Adv Exp Med Biol 2001; 496: 21-30.
[http://dx.doi.org/10.1007/978-1-4615-0651-5_3] [PMID: 11783621]

[109]   Eastell R, Lang T, Boonen S, *et al.* Effect of once-yearly zoledronic acid on the spine and hip as measured by quantitative computed tomography: results of the HORIZON Pivotal Fracture Trial. Osteoporos Int 2010; 21(7): 1277-85.
[http://dx.doi.org/10.1007/s00198-009-1077-9] [PMID: 19802508]

[110]   Genant HK, Engelke K, Hanley DA, *et al.* Denosumab improves density and strength parameters as measured by QCT of the radius in postmenopausal women with low bone mineral density. Bone 2010; 47(1): 131-9.
[http://dx.doi.org/10.1016/j.bone.2010.04.594] [PMID: 20399288]

[111]   Boutroy S, Van Rietbergen B, Sornay-Rendu E, Munoz F, Bouxsein ML, Delmas PD. Finite element analysis based on *in vivo* HR-pQCT images of the distal radius is associated with wrist fracture in postmenopausal women. J Bone Miner Res 2008; 23(3): 392-9.
[http://dx.doi.org/10.1359/jbmr.071108] [PMID: 17997712]

[112]   Vilayphiou N, Boutroy S, Szulc P, *et al.* Finite element analysis performed on radius and tibia HR-pQCT images and fragility fractures at all sites in men. J Bone Miner Res 2011; 26(5): 965-73.
[http://dx.doi.org/10.1002/jbmr.297] [PMID: 21541999]

[113] Ito M, Ejiri S, Jinnai H, *et al.* Bone structure and mineralization demonstrated using synchrotron radiation computed tomography (SR-CT) in animal models: preliminary findings. J Bone Miner Metab 2003; 21(5): 287-93.
[http://dx.doi.org/10.1007/s00774-003-0422-x] [PMID: 12928829]

[114] Borah B, Dufresne TE, Ritman EL, *et al.* Long-term risedronate treatment normalizes mineralization and continues to preserve trabecular architecture: sequential triple biopsy studies with micro-computed tomography. Bone 2006; 39(2): 345-52.
[http://dx.doi.org/10.1016/j.bone.2006.01.161] [PMID: 16571382]

[115] Peyrin F, Salome M, Cloetens P, Laval-Jeantet AM, Ritman E, Rüegsegger P. Micro-CT examinations of trabecular bone samples at different resolutions: 14, 7 and 2 micron level. Technol Health Care 1998; 6(5-6): 391-401.
[PMID: 10100941]

[116] Kinney JH, Lane NE, Haupt DL. *In vivo*, three-dimensional microscopy of trabecular bone. J Bone Miner Res 1995; 10(2): 264-70.
[http://dx.doi.org/10.1002/jbmr.5650100213] [PMID: 7754806]

[117] Kinney JH, Haupt DL, Balooch M, Ladd AJ, Ryaby JT, Lane NE. Three-dimensional morphometry of the L6 vertebra in the ovariectomized rat model of osteoporosis: biomechanical implications. J Bone Miner Res 2000; 15(10): 1981-91.
[http://dx.doi.org/10.1359/jbmr.2000.15.10.1981] [PMID: 11028451]

[118] Lane NE, Haupt D, Kimmel DB, Modin G, Kinney JH. Early estrogen replacement therapy reverses the rapid loss of trabecular bone volume and prevents further deterioration of connectivity in the rat. J Bone Miner Res 1999; 14(2): 206-14.
[http://dx.doi.org/10.1359/jbmr.1999.14.2.206] [PMID: 9933474]

[119] Lane NE, Thompson JM, Strewler GJ, Kinney JH. Intermittent treatment with human parathyroid hormone (hPTH[1-34]) increased trabecular bone volume but not connectivity in osteopenic rats. J Bone Miner Res 1995; 10(10): 1470-7.
[http://dx.doi.org/10.1002/jbmr.5650101007] [PMID: 8686502]

[120] Evans FG. Mechanical properties and histology of cortical bone from younger and older men. Anat Rec 1976; 185(1): 1-11.
[http://dx.doi.org/10.1002/ar.1091850102] [PMID: 1267192]

[121] Evans FG, Bang S. Differences and relationships between the physical properties and the microscopic structure of human femoral, tibial and fibular cortical bone. Am J Anat 1967; 120: 79-80.
[http://dx.doi.org/10.1002/aja.1001200107]

[122] Barth RW, Williams JL, Kaplan FS. Osteon morphometry in females with femoral neck fractures. Clin Orthop Relat Res 1992; (283): 178-86.
[PMID: 1395243]

[123] Skedros JG, Mason MW, Bloebaum RD. Differences in osteonal micromorphology between tensile and compressive cortices of a bending skeletal system: indications of potential strain-specific differences in bone microstructure. Anat Rec 1994; 239(4): 405-13.
[http://dx.doi.org/10.1002/ar.1092390407] [PMID: 7978364]

[124] Skedros JG, Mason MW, Nelson MC, Bloebaum RD. Evidence of structural and material adaptation to specific strain features in cortical bone. Anat Rec 1996; 246(1): 47-63.
[http://dx.doi.org/10.1002/(SICI)1097-0185(199609)246:1<47::AID-AR6>3.0.CO;2-C]   [PMID: 8876823]

[125] Mason MW, Skedros JG, Bloebaum RD. Evidence of strain-mode-related cortical adaptation in the diaphysis of the horse radius. Bone 1995; 17(3): 229-37.
[http://dx.doi.org/10.1016/8756-3282(95)00213-W] [PMID: 8541135]

[126] Currey JD. The effect of porosity and mineral content on the Young's modulus of elasticity of

compact bone. J Biomech 1988; 21(2): 131-9.
[http://dx.doi.org/10.1016/0021-9290(88)90006-1] [PMID: 3350827]

[127] Wachter NJ, Augat P, Krischak GD, *et al.* Prediction of strength of cortical bone in vitro by microcomputed tomography. Clin Biomech (Bristol, Avon) 2001; 16(3): 252-6.
[http://dx.doi.org/10.1016/S0268-0033(00)00092-9] [PMID: 11240061]

[128] Wehrli FW, Fernández-Seara MA. Nuclear magnetic resonance studies of bone water. Ann Biomed Eng 2005; 33(1): 79-86.
[http://dx.doi.org/10.1007/s10439-005-8965-8] [PMID: 15709708]

[129] Krug R, Larson PE, Wang C, *et al.* Ultrashort echo time MRI of cortical bone at 7 tesla field strength: a feasibility study. J Magn Reson Imaging 2011; 34(3): 691-5.
[http://dx.doi.org/10.1002/jmri.22648] [PMID: 21769960]

[130] Techawiboonwong A, Song HK, Leonard MB, Wehrli FW. Cortical bone water: *in vivo* quantification with ultrashort echo-time MR imaging. Radiology 2008; 248(3): 824-33.
[http://dx.doi.org/10.1148/radiol.2482071995] [PMID: 18632530]

[131] Currey JD. Effects of differences in mineralization on the mechanical properties of bone. Philos Trans R Soc Lond B Biol Sci 1984; 304(1121): 509-18.
[http://dx.doi.org/10.1098/rstb.1984.0042] [PMID: 6142490]

[132] An YH, Barfield WR, Knets I. Methods of evaluation for bone dimensions, densities, contents, morphology, and structuresMechanical testing of bone and the bone-implant interface. Boca Raton: CRC Press 2000; pp. 103-18.

[133] Paschalis EP, Glass EV, Donley DW, Eriksen EF. Bone mineral and collagen quality in iliac crest biopsies of patients given teriparatide: new results from the fracture prevention trial. J Clin Endocrinol Metab 2005; 90(8): 4644-9.
[http://dx.doi.org/10.1210/jc.2004-2489] [PMID: 15914535]

[134] Faibish D, Gomes A, Boivin G, Binderman I, Boskey A. Infrared imaging of calcified tissue in bone biopsies from adults with osteomalacia. Bone 2005; 36(1): 6-12.
[http://dx.doi.org/10.1016/j.bone.2004.08.019] [PMID: 15663997]

[135] Camacho NP, Carroll P, Raggio CL. Fourier transform infrared imaging spectroscopy (FT-IRIS) of mineralization in bisphosphonate-treated oim/oim mice. Calcif Tissue Int 2003; 72(5): 604-9.
[http://dx.doi.org/10.1007/s00223-002-1038-1] [PMID: 12574874]

[136] Akkus O, Polyakova-Akkus A, Adar F, Schaffler MB. Aging of microstructural compartments in human compact bone. J Bone Miner Res 2003; 18(6): 1012-9.
[http://dx.doi.org/10.1359/jbmr.2003.18.6.1012] [PMID: 12817753]

[137] Qin L, Hung L, Leung K, Guo X, Bumrerraj S, Katz L. Staining intensity of individual osteons correlated with elastic properties and degrees of mineralization. J Bone Miner Metab 2001; 19(6): 359-64.
[http://dx.doi.org/10.1007/s007740170005] [PMID: 11685651]

[138] Qin L, Bumrerraj S, Leung K, Katz L. Correlation study of scanning acoustic microscope reflection coefficients and image brightness intensities of micrographed osteons. J Bone Miner Metab 2004; 22(2): 86-9.
[http://dx.doi.org/10.1007/s00774-003-0454-2] [PMID: 14999517]

[139] Vajda EG, Skedros JG, Bloebaum RD. Consistency in calibrated backscattered electron images of calcified tissues and minerals analyzed in multiple imaging sessions. Scanning Microsc 1995; 9(3): 741-53.
[PMID: 9565522]

[140] Bachus KN, Bloebaum RD. Projection effect errors in biomaterials and bone research. Cells Mater 1992; 2(4): 347-55.

[141] Roschger P, Rinnerthaler S, Yates J, Rodan GA, Fratzl P, Klaushofer K. Alendronate increases degree

and uniformity of mineralization in cancellous bone and decreases the porosity in cortical bone of osteoporotic women. Bone 2001; 29(2): 185-91.
[http://dx.doi.org/10.1016/S8756-3282(01)00485-9] [PMID: 11502482]

[142] Borah B, Ritman EL, Dufresne TE, *et al.* The effect of risedronate on bone mineralization as measured by micro-computed tomography with synchrotron radiation: correlation to histomorphometric indices of turnover. Bone 2005; 37(1): 1-9.
[http://dx.doi.org/10.1016/j.bone.2005.03.017] [PMID: 15894527]

[143] Vajda EG, Humphrey S, Skedros JG, Bloebaum RD. Influence of topography and specimen preparation on backscattered electron images of bone. Scanning 1999; 21(6): 379-87.
[http://dx.doi.org/10.1002/sca.4950210604] [PMID: 10654424]

[144] Martin RB, Ishida J. The relative effects of collagen fiber orientation, porosity, density, and mineralization on bone strength. J Biomech 1989; 22(5): 419-26.
[http://dx.doi.org/10.1016/0021-9290(89)90202-9] [PMID: 2777816]

[145] Martin RB, Boardman DL. The effects of collagen fiber orientation, porosity, density, and mineralization on bovine cortical bone bending properties. J Biomech 1993; 26(9): 1047-54.
[http://dx.doi.org/10.1016/S0021-9290(05)80004-1] [PMID: 8408087]

[146] Meunier PJ, Boivin G. Bone mineral density reflects bone mass but also the degree of mineralization of bone: therapeutic implications. Bone 1997; 21(5): 373-7.
[http://dx.doi.org/10.1016/S8756-3282(97)00170-1] [PMID: 9356729]

[147] Boivin GY, Chavassieux PM, Santora AC, Yates J, Meunier PJ. Alendronate increases bone strength by increasing the mean degree of mineralization of bone tissue in osteoporotic women. Bone 2000; 27(5): 687-94.
[http://dx.doi.org/10.1016/S8756-3282(00)00376-8] [PMID: 11062357]

[148] Huang TH, Lin SC, Chang FL, Hsieh SS, Liu SH, Yang RS. Effects of different exercise modes on mineralization, structure, and biomechanical properties of growing bone. J Appl Physiol 2003; 95(1): 300-7.
[http://dx.doi.org/10.1152/japplphysiol.01076.2002] [PMID: 12611764]

[149] Follet H, Boivin G, Rumelhart C, Meunier PJ. The degree of mineralization is a determinant of bone strength: a study on human calcanei. Bone 2004; 34(5): 783-9.
[http://dx.doi.org/10.1016/j.bone.2003.12.012] [PMID: 15121009]

[150] Carando S, Portigliatti Barbos M, Ascenzi A, Boyde A. Orientation of collagen in human tibial and fibular shaft and possible correlation with mechanical properties. Bone 1989; 10(2): 139-42.
[http://dx.doi.org/10.1016/8756-3282(89)90012-4] [PMID: 2765311]

[151] Boyde A, Riggs CM. The quantitative study of the orientation of collagen in compact bone slices. Bone 1990; 11(1): 35-9.
[http://dx.doi.org/10.1016/8756-3282(90)90069-B] [PMID: 2331429]

[152] Martin RB, Lau ST, Mathews PV, Gibson VA, Stover SM. Collagen fiber organization is related to mechanical properties and remodeling in equine bone. A comparison of two methods. J Biomech 1996; 29(12): 1515-21.
[http://dx.doi.org/10.1016/S0021-9290(96)80002-9] [PMID: 8945649]

[153] Skedros JG. Collagen fiber orientation: A characteristics of strain-mode-related regional adaptation in cortical bone. Bone 2001; 28: s110-1.

[154] Skedros JG, *et al.* The influence of collagen fiber orientation on mechanical properties of cortical bone of an artiodactyl calcaneus: Implications for broad applications in bone adaptation. Trans Orthop Res Soc 2003; 28: 411.

[155] Riggs CM, Lanyon LE, Boyde A. Functional associations between collagen fibre orientation and locomotor strain direction in cortical bone of the equine radius. Anat Embryol (Berl) 1993; 187(3): 231-8.

[PMID: 8470823]

[156] Carando S, Portigliatti-Barbos M, Ascenzi A, Riggs CM, Boyde A. Macroscopic shape of, and lamellar distribution within, the upper limb shafts, allowing inferences about mechanical properties. Bone 1991; 12(4): 265-9.
[http://dx.doi.org/10.1016/8756-3282(91)90074-S] [PMID: 1793677]

[157] Skedros JG, Dayton MR, Bachus KN. Strain-mode specific loading of cortical bone reveals important role for collagen fiber orientation in energy absorption. Trans Orthop Res Soc 2001; 26: 519.

[158] Pearson OM, Lieberman DE. The aging of Wolff's "law": ontogeny and responses to mechanical loading in cortical bone. Am J Phys Anthropol 2004; (Suppl. 39)63-99.
[http://dx.doi.org/10.1002/ajpa.20155] [PMID: 15605390]

[159] Schaffler MB, Choi K, Milgrom C. Aging and matrix microdamage accumulation in human compact bone. Bone 1995; 17(6): 521-5.
[http://dx.doi.org/10.1016/8756-3282(95)00370-3] [PMID: 8835305]

[160] Burr DB, Forwood MR, Fyhrie DP, Martin RB, Schaffler MB, Turner CH. Bone microdamage and skeletal fragility in osteoporotic and stress fractures. J Bone Miner Res 1997; 12(1): 6-15.
[http://dx.doi.org/10.1359/jbmr.1997.12.1.6] [PMID: 9240720]

[161] Vashishth D, Koontz J, Qiu SJ, *et al.* *In vivo* diffuse damage in human vertebral trabecular bone. Bone 2000; 26(2): 147-52.
[http://dx.doi.org/10.1016/S8756-3282(99)00253-7] [PMID: 10678409]

[162] Burr DB, Turner CH, Naick P, *et al.* Does microdamage accumulation affect the mechanical properties of bone? J Biomech 1998; 31(4): 337-45.
[http://dx.doi.org/10.1016/S0021-9290(98)00016-5] [PMID: 9672087]

[163] Schaffler MB, Radin EL, Burr DB. Long-term fatigue behavior of compact bone at low strain magnitude and rate. Bone 1990; 11(5): 321-6.
[http://dx.doi.org/10.1016/8756-3282(90)90087-F] [PMID: 2252810]

[164] Pattin CA, Caler WE, Carter DR. Cyclic mechanical property degradation during fatigue loading of cortical bone. J Biomech 1996; 29(1): 69-79.
[http://dx.doi.org/10.1016/0021-9290(94)00156-1] [PMID: 8839019]

[165] Zioupos P, Wang XT, Currey JD. The accumulation of fatigue microdamage in human cortical bone of two different ages *in vitro.* Clin Biomech (Bristol, Avon) 1996; 11(7): 365-75.
[http://dx.doi.org/10.1016/0268-0033(96)00010-1] [PMID: 11415648]

[166] Carter DR, Hayes WC. Compact bone fatigue damage-I. Residual strength and stiffness. J Biomech 1977; 10(5-6): 325-37.
[http://dx.doi.org/10.1016/0021-9290(77)90005-7] [PMID: 893471]

[167] Mori S, Burr DB. Increased intracortical remodeling following fatigue damage. Bone 1993; 14(2): 103-9.
[http://dx.doi.org/10.1016/8756-3282(93)90235-3] [PMID: 8334026]

[168] Qiu S, Rao DS, Fyhrie DP, Palnitkar S, Parfitt AM. The morphological association between microcracks and osteocyte lacunae in human cortical bone. Bone 2005; 37(1): 10-5.
[http://dx.doi.org/10.1016/j.bone.2005.01.023] [PMID: 15878702]

CHAPTER 8

Computer-Aided Diagnosis Model for Skin Cancer Detection

Abstract: This chapter introduces a computer-aided method to detect skin lesion using image features and shape features. Artificial neural networks (ANNs) trained with image features (energy, contrast, homogeneity and correlation) and shape features (asymmetry, border irregularity, color and diameter) in differentiating common nevus, atypical nevus and melanoma using dermoscopy images were described. 120 dermoscopy skin lesion images were collected from online PH2 database. The model was built on a single 3 layers, feed forward back propagation ANNs trained and tested with round robin method. The ANN's performance was evaluated with receiver operating characteristic (ROC) analysis and chi-square test. The performance was evaluated by comparing total dermoscopy score method with ANNs method. Our result noted that the area under curve (Az) of ROC were 0.807 for differentiating atypical nevus from common nevus, 0.998 for differentiating melanoma from common nevus and 0.959 for i differentiating melanoma from atypical nevus, respectively. This indicated that the ANNs method provided an accurate differential diagnosis in common skin lesions for dermoscopy images.

1. INTRODUCTION

Skin cancer is one of the common cancers in the world that is mainly caused by ultraviolet radiation and genetics [1]. Basal cell carcinoma, squamous cell carcinoma and melanoma are three most common type of skin cancer that responsible for 99% of skin cancers [2]. Basal cell carcinoma and squamous cell carcinoma are less dangerous as they rarely metastasize to other parts of the body. However, melanoma is more aggressive and metastatic. 75% of mortality in skin cancers is resulted from melanoma. It arises from the melanocytes, which can appear as new color spot or a change in appearance of the skin. Melanoma could be misclassified as nevi, which are formed because of the neoplasia and hyperplasia of melanocytes [3]. Dysplastic nevi appears larger in size with irregular and indistinct borders, and has the potential to grow into melanoma.

The current method of diagnosing skin cancer is by visual inspection by a dermatologist [4]. Dermatoscopy is commonly used to aid visualizing the morphological features of the melanomas by magnification. However, the accuracy of dermoscopic examination relies heavily on the examiner. Skilled dermatologist can achieve 90% sensitivity and 59% specificity, while junior doctors could only attain 62% sensitivity [5]. Skin biopsy is an accurate method, but it is time consuming and could cause complications such as bleeding and tumor cell seeding [6]. The 5-year survival rates would drop significantly from 94.1% to 4.6% if the malignant melanoma are detected in stage 4 rather than stage 1, due to likelihood of distant metastases. Thus early diagnosis of melanoma can greatly improved prognosis as the cancer can be removed completely without complications [7].

Artificial neural networks (ANNs) have been used to provide objective measurement and reduce the false negative rates of clinical practitioner when interpreting medical images [8]. ANNs which simulate human neural networks, have been recently adopted in the early diagnosis of melanoma [9]. In previous studies, grey level co-occurrence matrix features and clinical features have been taken into the training and testing of ANN, with an accuracy ranging from 80%-92% [9 - 12].

In this chapter, we describe an ANNs method to differentiate diagnosis of common nevus, atypical nevus and melanoma on dermoscopic images.

2. MATERIALS AND METHODS

2.1. Image Acquisition

200 images were collected from the PH2 dermatoscopy online database, which contained dermatoscopy images (20x magnification) obtained at the Dermatology Service of Hospital Pedro Hispano. The skin lesions collected have been diagnosed by dermatologists, including 80 common nevi, 80 atypical nevi and 40 melanomas. The images were acquired with 8-bit color images with 768x560 resolution.

2.2. Image Processing and Features Extraction

2.2.1. Image Preprocessing

The image was firstly preprocessed to remove unwanted signal or noise and to enhance the important features [13] and resized to a consistent dimension (800x800 pixels). The area-of-interest (ROI) was selected manually where the image features (energy, contrast, homogeneity and correlation) based on grey level co-occurrence matrix (GLCM) [14, 15] and lesion shape features (asymmetry, border irregularity, color and diameter) were extracted (Fig. **1**).

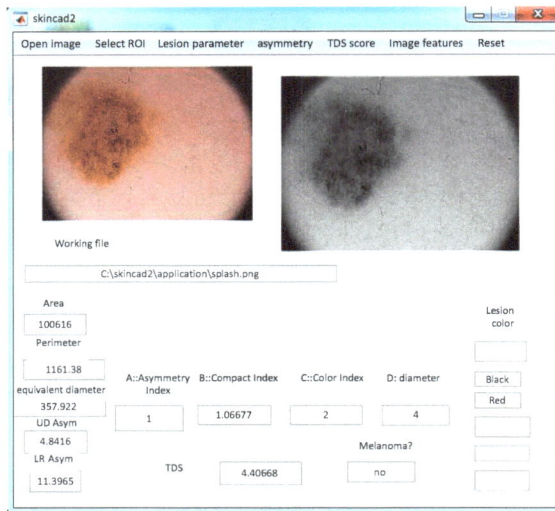

Fig. (1). Interface of the feature extraction program.

2.2.2. Image Segmentation

Manual segmentation was performed to locate the boundaries of the skin lesions and remove unnecessary signal and noise (Fig. **2**). Intra-class Correlation Coefficient (ICC) was performed to test the reliability of operator's segmentation.

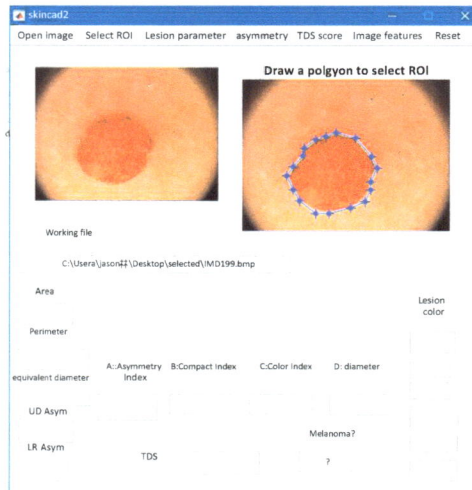

Fig. (2). Selection of ROI of skin.

2.3. Image and Lesion Shape Features Calculation

There were eight features selected for the detection of skin cancer used for ANNs, these included: energy, contrast, homogeneity, correlation, asymmetry, border irregularity, color, and diameter.

Energy, contrast, homogeneity and correlation were calculated based on Gray Level Co-occurrence Matrix parameters for features extraction [16]. The image features were calculated by the Texture Analysis using Gray-Level Co-Occurrence Matrix given by Matlab

(https://www.mathworks.com/help/images/texture-analysis-using-the-gray-level-co-occurrence-matrix-glcm.html;jsessionid=aef286901604bb42df7b7e023aa5?s_tid=gn_loc_drop)

The skin lesion features were: asymmetry, border irregularity, color, diameter and total dermoscopy score. These were clinical features based on the ABCD rule of dermoscopy developed by dermatologist and were considered important parameters for the diagnosis of melanoma clinically [17]. Melanoma is often asymmetric, while common nevi is usually symmetrical. Melanoma tends to be ill-defined with irregular borders. It may contain different colors such as blue, black and brown. The diameter of melanoma is often longer and exceeded 6 millimeters.

In order to calculate the asymmetry index, the skin lesion was bisected by a vertical axis and horizontal axis. The area difference between the bisected portions was calculated by the following formula [17],

$$AI = \frac{\Delta A}{A} \times 100$$

A= Area of the lesion. ΔA= Area difference between the bisected portions

When the area difference between the two areas was >5%, it was considered as asymmetric. If both axes were asymmetric, the asymmetry score was 2. If there was asymmetry on one axis only, the score was 1. If the lesion was symmetric in the two axes, the score was 0. The calculation of asymmetry was illustrated in Fig. (**3**).

Border irregularity was calculated using compact index (CI. Irregular object would have a higher compact index value. Its value ranged 0 to 8. The calculation of compact index is given by [17]:

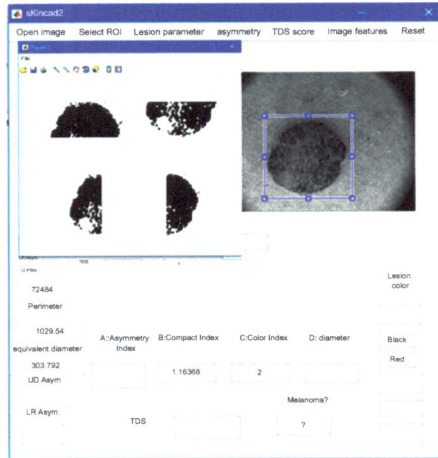

Fig. (3). Illustration of asymmetry calculation.

$$CI = \frac{P_L^2}{4\pi A_L}$$ P_L = Perimeter of the Lesion. A_L = Area of the Lesion.

For the color index, white, red, light brown, dark brown, blue-gray, and black were the six color that would be detected and recorded. Presence of each color would contribute to one color score, which range from 0-6. A color that accounted for more than 10% of the total pixel number of the image would be counted. The RGB color space for the six color mention was illustrated in Table **1** [17]:

Table 1. RGB to grayscale conversion table.

Color	RGB	rgb
White	255,255,255	1.0,1.0,1.0
Black	0,0,0	0.0,0.0,0.0
Red	255,0,0	1.0,0.0,0.0
Light Brown	205,133,63	0.80,0.52,0.25
Dark Brown	101,67,33	0.40,0.26,0.13
Blue Gray	0,134,139	0.0,0.52,0.54

The diameter was measured manually, by taking the average between vertical and horizontal diameter of the lesion.

Total dermoscopy score based on the asymmetry, border irregularity, color and diameter of the lesion, with TDS = Asymmetry*1.3 + Border irregularity *0.1 +

Color*0.5 + Diameter*0.5. The maximum score of TDS was 8.9, score <4.75 was classified as common nevus, 4.8-5.45 as atypical nevus, >5.45 as melanoma.

2.4. Artificial Neural Networks

This study implemented a single three-layer ANNs using feed forward back propagation algorithm. The advantage of using ANNs was that it had the ability to analyze and solve complex data with the nonlinear processing capabilities of ANNs neurons [18]. Back propagation was the method for the training of the artificial neural networks [19]. The algorithm consisted of two main flows, which were propagation and weight update. Every input feature to the ANNs would be propagated in the forward direction forward through the input layer, hidden layer and output layer. Then a loss function would be used to compare the output of ANNs with the desired output, generating an error value. This error value would be propagated backwards and weighting of both hidden and output layer would be adjusted until the error becomes zero.

The ANNs were developed for the differentiation of common nevus, atypical nevus and melanoma by using 4 Gray Level Co-occurrence Matrix features (energy, contrast, homogeneity and correlation) and ABCD features (asymmetry, border irregularity, color and diameter) as input unit. As a result, the ANN consisted of 8 input units and 1 output unit that ranged from 0 to 2 that represented the differential diagnosis (common nevus=0, atypical nevus =1 and melanoma=2). The amount of hidden units was determined by the ANNs. The structure of ANN was illustrated by Fig. (**4**).

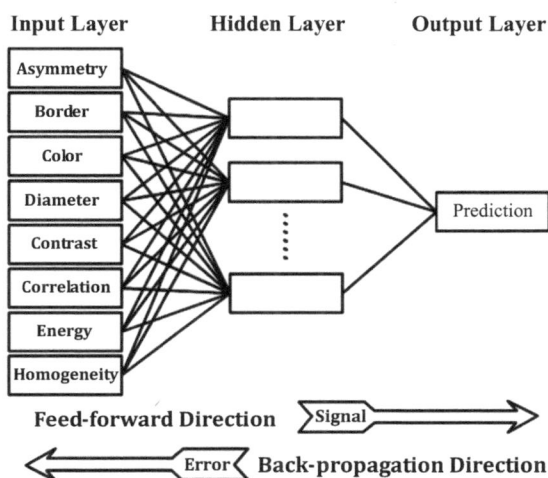

Fig. (4). Illustration of ANN structure.

Round robin method was used for the training and testing of the ANN in the performance evaluation of the merged features. The ANN was trained on the 8 features mentioned above for each training image and the result of the testing image was compared with the true diagnosis. Therefore, the ANN was trained and tested on a per-image basis. We trained and tested the ANNs using the Round Robin or leave-one- out method where 1 case was selected for test and the rest were used for training repeatedly until all the images in the database would be used once as a testing case, *i.e.* 120 times repeated for 120 images [20].

2.5. Data Analysis

Intra-class Correlation Coefficient (ICC) was performed to test the reliability of operator's manual segmentation of skin lesions. 8 images were randomly selected and manual segmentations were performed 5 times each by 6 assessors. ICC Model 2 is used for testing intra-rater reliability and ICC Model 3 for inter-rater reliability (IBM SPSS Statistics 23 is used).

DeLong *et al.*'s method was used for the ROC data analysis using MedCalc statistical software [21].

The diagnostic performance of ANN and TDS system were evaluated by ROC analysis. Three categories of ROC curves were generated, which include the diagnosis of common nevus against atypical nevus, common nevus against melanoma and atypical nevus against melanoma. The ANN's performance was compared with total dermoscopy score by calculating the standard score between the ROC curves of ANN and total dermoscopy score.

3. RESULTS

Our ICC test indicated a good reliability (average intraclass correlation =0.994, interclass correlation=0.884) among 6 different assessors of images using manual segmentation of skin lesions (Table **2**).

Table 2. ICC test for reliability.

Assessor	Intraclass Correlation
Intraclass Correlation for 6 assessors	0.994
Interclass Correlation for 6 assessors	0.884

120 images from the PH2 database (40 common nevi, 40 atypical nevi and 40 melanomas) were obtained. ROC analysis was performed to evaluate the performance of ANN in the differential diagnosis of common nevus, atypical nevus and melanoma.

The performance of artificial neural network and total dermoscopy score in differentiating atypical nevus from common nevus, melanoma from common nevus and melanoma from atypical nevus using ROC analysis was demonstrated in the Fig. (**1**). Table **3** summarized the ROC results of the performance of artificial neural network (ANN) and total dermoscopy score (TDS).

On the whole, artificial neural network significantly performed better then TDS system ($p < 0.05$, chi-square test), except in differentiating atypical nevus from common nevus ($p > 0.05$, chi square test, Table **4**).

Table 3. ROC results of the performance of artificial neural network and total dermoscopy score.

	Differentiating Atypical Nevus from Common Nevus	Differentiating Melanoma from Common Nevus	Differentiating Melanoma from Atypical Nevus
ANN method	Az =0.807	Az =0.998	Az =0.959
TDS method	Az =0.7	Az =0.863	Az =0.709

The overall accuracy of ANN method was 80%. Table **5** showed the sensitivity and specificity of ANN method in differentiating atypical nevus from common nevus, melanoma from common nevus and melanoma from atypical nevus.

Table 4. Performance of ANNs with TDS for differentiation different skin lesions (chi square test).

Differentiating melanoma from atypical nevus with ANNs and TDS	P<0.0001
Differentiating melanoma from common nevus with ANNs and TDS.	P<0.001
Differentiating atypical nevus from common nevus with ANNs and TDS score.	p>0.05

Table 5. Sensitivity and specificity of ANNs method.

	Differentiating Atypical Nevus from Common Nevus	Differentiating Melanoma from Common Nevus	Differentiating Melanoma from Atypical Nevus
Sensitivity	75%	80%	80%
Specificity	85%	85%	75%

4. DISCUSSION

Performance of Artificial Neural Networks System for Skin Lesion Detection

Our result indicated that when combining image textual features (Gray Level Co-occurrence Matrix features: energy, contrast, homogeneity and correlation) with shape features (ABCD features: asymmetry, border irregularity, color and diameter), good performance of the ANNs system for differentiating skin lesions was obtained. In terms of diagnostic accuracy, ANNs method achieved 85% for common nevus, 75% for atypical nevus and 80% for melanoma. The performance of artificial neural network was comparable to similar results (80-92% accuracy) using computer aided detection of melanoma [9 - 12].

When comparing with TDS score method alone, ANNs method had a better diagnostic accuracy in differentiating common nevus, atypical nevus and melanoma. The Az values in ANN were generally higher than that of TDS system (Table **3**). On the whole, there are significant difference in performance for ANNs method when comparing with TDS method ($p < 0.05$) except in differentiating atypical nevus from common nevus (Table **4**).

Comparison with Previous Studies

In former studies, only GLCM image features, but not ABCD features, were taken for the training of artificial neural network [22 - 28]. Garnavi *et al.* [29] used 23 borders and wavelet-based image textures for CAD of melanoma, and achieved an accuracy of 91.26% with AUC value of 0.937 and their performance was comparable with ours (88.75% accuracy). In their study, they used 4 classifiers, (Support Vector Machine, Random Forest, Logistic Model Tree and Hidden Naive Bayes) while our method appeared to be simple and straightforward.

FURTHER CONSIDERATIONS

Previous study showed that junior doctors could only achieve 62% sensitivity in diagnosing melanoma [5]. Our ANNs system performed better with 88.75% accuracy. This computer aided diagnosis based on image processing technique can act as a reference guidance that junior/frontline doctors.

With the rapid growth of smart devices, it is possible to combine this ANNs method to analyze image taken from individual using micro-lens attached to smartphones, where skin images can be uploaded and analysed with online cloud service. Then the images could be input to the ANN and generate the diagnosis of skin lesions. Thus a smartphone app can be developed for this purpose in the future applications.

CONCLUSION

This chapter illustrates the incorporation of Gray Level Co-occurrence Matrix features and ABCD features in training of an ANNs system. The ANNs could provide an accurate differential diagnosis in common nevus, atypical nevus and melanoma using dermoscopy images.

REFERENCES

[1]   Heim S, Mitelman F. Cancer cytogenetics: chromosomal and molecular genetic aberrations of tumor cells. John Wiley & Sons 2015; pp. 57-9.
[http://dx.doi.org/10.1002/9781118795569]

[2]   Lomas A, Leonardi-Bee J, Bath-Hextall F. A systematic review of worldwide incidence of nonmelanoma skin cancer. Br J Dermatol 2012; 166(5): 1069-80.
[http://dx.doi.org/10.1111/j.1365-2133.2012.10830.x] [PMID: 22251204]

[3]   Goldstein AM, Tucker MA. Dysplastic nevi and melanoma. Cancer Epidemiol Biomarkers Prev 2013; 22(4): 528-32.
[http://dx.doi.org/10.1158/1055-9965.EPI-12-1346] [PMID: 23549396]

[4]   Vestergaard ME, Macaskill P, Holt PE, Menzies SW. Dermoscopy compared with naked eye examination for the diagnosis of primary melanoma: a meta-analysis of studies performed in a clinical setting. Br J Dermatol 2008; 159(3): 669-76.
[PMID: 18616769]

[5]   Menzies SW, Bischof L, Talbot H, *et al.* The performance of SolarScan: an automated dermoscopy image analysis instrument for the diagnosis of primary melanoma. Arch Dermatol 2005; 141(11): 1388-96.
[http://dx.doi.org/10.1001/archderm.141.11.1388] [PMID: 16301386]

[6]   Hardenbergh G. Rapid diagnosis of acute meningococcal infections by needle aspiration or biopsy of skin lesions. Ann Emerg Med 1993; 22: 1642-3.
[http://dx.doi.org/10.1016/S0196-0644(05)81284-3]

[7]   Chi Z, Li S, Sheng X, *et al.* Clinical presentation, histology, and prognoses of malignant melanoma in ethnic Chinese: a study of 522 consecutive cases. BMC Cancer 2011; 11: 85.
[http://dx.doi.org/10.1186/1471-2407-11-85] [PMID: 21349197]

[8]   Abe H, Ashizawa K, Katsuragawa S, MacMahon H, Doi K. Use of an artificial neural network to determine the diagnostic value of specific clinical and radiologic parameters in the diagnosis of interstitial lung disease on chest radiographs. Acad Radiol 2002; 9(1): 13-7.
[http://dx.doi.org/10.1016/S1076-6332(03)80291-X] [PMID: 11918354]

[9]   Masood A, Al-Jumaily AA. Computer aided diagnostic support system for skin cancer: a review of techniques and algorithms. Int J Biomed Imaging 2013; 2013: 323268.
[http://dx.doi.org/10.1155/2013/323268] [PMID: 24575126]

[10]   Bhuiyan M, Azad I, Uddin M. Image processing for skin cancer features extraction. Int J Sci Eng Res 2013; 4: 1-6.

[11]   Jain S, Jagtap V, Pise N. Computer Aided Melanoma Skin Cancer Detection Using Image Processing. Procedia Comput Sci 2015; 48: 735-40.
[http://dx.doi.org/10.1016/j.procs.2015.04.209]

[12]   Amaliah B, Fatichah C, Widyanto M. ABCD feature extraction of image dermatoscopic based on morphology analysis for melanoma skin cancer diagnosis. Jurnal Ilmu Komputer dan Informasi 2012; 3: 82-90.

[13]   Saha S, Gupta R. An Automated Skin Lesion Diagnosis by using Image Processing Techniques. International Journal on Recent and Innovation Trends in Computing and Communication 2014; 2: 1081-5.

[14]   Guyon I, Elisseeff A. An introduction to feature extraction.Feature extraction. Springer Berlin Heidelberg 2006; pp. 1-15.
[http://dx.doi.org/10.1007/978-3-540-35488-8_1]

[15]   Guo J, Menon PG. Feature Based Classification of Melanoma from Skin Images. American Society of Mechanical Engineers 2015; p. 83.
[http://dx.doi.org/10.1115/IMECE2015-50055]

[16]   Sheha MA, Mabrouk MS, Sharawy A. Automatic detection of melanoma skin cancer using texture analysis. Int J Comput Appl 2012; 42: 22-6.

[17]   She Z, Liu Y, Damatoa A. Combination of features from skin pattern and ABCD analysis for lesion classification. Skin Res Technol 2007; 13(1): 25-33.
[http://dx.doi.org/10.1111/j.1600-0846.2007.00181.x] [PMID: 17250529]

[18]   Lisboa PJ, Taktak AF. The use of artificial neural networks in decision support in cancer: a systematic review. Neural Netw 2006; 19(4): 408-15.
[http://dx.doi.org/10.1016/j.neunet.2005.10.007] [PMID: 16483741]

[19]   Graupe D. Principles of artificial neural networks. World Scientific 2013; pp. 1-20.
[http://dx.doi.org/10.1142/8868]

[20]   Fürnkranz J. Round robin classification. J Mach Learn Res 2002; 2: 721-47.

[21]   Hajian-Tilaki K. Receiver operating characteristic (ROC) curve analysis for medical diagnostic test evaluation. Caspian J Intern Med 2013; 4(2): 627-35.
[PMID: 24009950]

[22]   Clausi DA. An analysis of co-occurrence texture statistics as a function of grey level quantization. Can J Rem Sens 2002; 28: 45-62.
[http://dx.doi.org/10.5589/m02-004]

[23]   Ruiz D, Berenguer V, Soriano A, Sanchez B. A decision ´ support system for the diagnosis of melanoma: a comparative approach. Expert Syst Appl 2011; 32: 15217-23.
[http://dx.doi.org/10.1016/j.eswa.2011.05.079]

[24]   Lee TK, McLean DI, Atkins MS. Irregularity index: a new border irregularity measure for cutaneous melanocytic lesions. Med Image Anal 2003; 7(1): 47-64.
[http://dx.doi.org/10.1016/S1361-8415(02)00090-7] [PMID: 12467721]

[25]   Claridge E, Hall PN, Keefe M, Allen JP. Shape analysis for classification of malignant melanoma. J Biomed Eng 1992; 14(3): 229-34.
[http://dx.doi.org/10.1016/0141-5425(92)90057-R] [PMID: 1588780]

[26]   Ercal F, Chawla A, Stoecker WV, Lee HC, Moss RH. Neural network diagnosis of malignant melanoma from color images. IEEE Trans Biomed Eng 1994; 41(9): 837-45.
[http://dx.doi.org/10.1109/10.312091] [PMID: 7959811]

[27]   Schmid-Saugeon P. Symmetry axis computation for almost-symmetrical and asymmetrical objects: application to pigmented skin lesions. Med Image Anal 2000; 4(3): 269-82.
[http://dx.doi.org/10.1016/S1361-8415(00)00019-0] [PMID: 11145313]

[28]   Stoecker WV, Wronkiewiecz M, Chowdhury R, *et al*. Detection of granularity in dermoscopy images of malignant melanoma using color and texture features. Comput Med Imaging Graph 2011; 35(2): 144-7.
[http://dx.doi.org/10.1016/j.compmedimag.2010.09.005] [PMID: 21036538]

[29]   Garnavi R, Aldeen M, Bailey J. Computer-aided diagnosis of melanoma using border and wavelet-based texture analysis. IEEE Trans Inf Technol Biomed 2012; 16(6): 1239-52.
[http://dx.doi.org/10.1109/TITB.2012.2212282] [PMID: 22893445]

SUBJECT INDEX

A

Adaptive partial smoothing filter (APSF) 27
Advanced imaging sequence 65
Affine transformation 37, 40
Alendronate 68
APOE alleles 47, 48
Artificial neural network (ANNs) 26, 28, 30, 31, 32, 83, 84, 86, 88, 89, 90, 91
Artificial neural networks 28, 83, 84, 88, 90, 91
Asymmetry calculation 86, 87
Asymptomatic patients 15
Atypical nevus 83, 84, 88, 89, 90, 91

B

Backscattered electrons 65, 67
Basal cell carcinoma 83
Beam hardening effect 60, 61, 66
Big data analytics 15, 17, 18
Binarized image 58
Biomechanical breast model 42
Birefringent effect 69
BMD measurements 56, 58, 61
Bone adaptation 53
Bone density 55, 57, 63
Bone marrow 58, 59
Bone matrix 65, 67
Bone micro-architecture 56, 57, 66
Bone mineralization 65, 66, 67
Bone modelling 53, 54
Bone quality 53, 59, 63
Bone quantity 53, 63
Bone specimen 67, 69
Bone status 53, 64, 71
Bone strength 53, 54, 55, 63, 67
Bone structure 56
Border irregularity 83, 84, 86, 87, 88, 90
Boundary conditions 38, 39
Brain imaging data sequences ranging 46

Brain volume 49
Breast cancer 15, 35, 36, 42
Breast deformation 37, 39
Breast images 36, 37, 40
Breast Modeling 35
Broadband ultrasound attenuation (BUA) 55, 56
BSE images 65

C

CAD component 3, 10
CAD METHOD 27
CAD system 26, 30, 31, 32
CAD System by Model Observer 30
Calcaneum 55, 56, 58
CAROI method 28, 29
Cerebro-spinal fluid (CSF) 46, 47, 48
Channelized hotelling observer (CHO) 30, 31
Circular adaptive region of interest (CAROI) 28, 29
Circular adaptive regions 28
Circularly polarized light (CPL) 53, 68, 69
Clinical risk factors 56
Cloud computing 1, 2, 6, 10, 31
Cloud technology 2, 7, 10, 12
Clustering of APOE alleles 47, 48, 51
Cognitive function 45, 46
Cognitive status 48, 49
Cognitive systems 22
Collagen fibre orientation (CFO) 68, 69
Collagen fibres 53, 54, 68, 69
Common nevus 83, 84, 86, 88, 89, 90, 91
 diagnosis of 84, 89
 differentiating 83, 91
Components 2, 3, 8, 9, 10, 47, 53, 66
 file management 8, 9
 image importer 8, 9
 image processor 8
Composite tissue 53
Compression cortex 69, 70

Isotropic voxel size 61, 62

J

Joint endplate 58

L

Large-scale deformation 35
Leave-one-out method 30
Lesion diameter 40
Light, polarized 68, 69

M

Magnetic axes 57
    field, external 57
Magnetic resonance imaging (MRI) 7, 15, 20,
        27, 35, 36, 39, 45, 53, 57, 64
Material properties 36, 39, 54
    initial 39
Mean decrease 19, 21
    accuracy (MDA) 19, 21
    Gini (MDG) 19
Mechanical properties 39, 62, 65, 68, 70
Medical application 6, 35, 51
Medical fields 6, 14, 16
Medical images 6, 7, 14, 15, 26, 84
    interpreting 84
Medical imaging examinations 22
Melanocytes 83
Melanoma 83, 84, 86, 88, 89, 90, 91
    diagnosing 91
    early diagnosis of 84
Micro-architecture 54, 63, 67
Microdamage 53, 70
    morphology 70
Microradiographic images 66
Mild cognitive impairment (MCI) 45, 47, 48,
        49, 50
Mobile application client 6, 7, 8, 11
Mobile application server 6, 7, 8
    core program 8
Mobile devices 1, 3, 7, 8, 10, 11, 12, 31
    smart 1, 3

Mobile PACS 6, 7
Mobile phone 6, 7, 9, 11
Mobile technology 7, 10, 31
Mobile web interface 7
Modalities 15, 53, 56
    multi-imaging 53
Modality performed procedure step (MPPS)
        17
Model 35, 36, 39, 41, 42
    deformed 39
    mechanical 35, 41, 42
    registration 35, 36
Morphologic parameters 58
MRI breast images 35
MRI images 36
MR image quality 58
MR images 36, 37, 40, 46, 57, 58, 59, 6
    acquired 58
    calcaneal 59
    collected 46
    high resolution 58, 60
MR imaging 58, 59, 60, 65
    dynamic contrast-enhanced 60
    ultra-short echo time 65
MR imaging techniques 59
MRI scans 36
MR Registration 35, 36
Multi-modality imaging methods 71
Multiple decision trees 19
Multi-slice spiral CT 60, 61

N

Network connections 1
Neurological disorder 45
NeuroQuant 49, 50
    report 49, 50
Node impurities 19
Non-contrast sagittal images 49
Non-mechanical factors 53, 54

O

Optical transmission axis 69
Orthopaedics 55, 61, 62, 63, 64